D1611979

LAPAROSCOPY FOR GYNECOLOGY AND ONCOLOGY

PROCEDURES DVD AND MANUAL

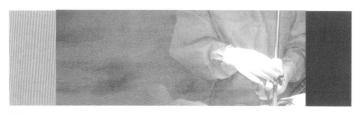

LAPAROSCOPY FOR GYNECOLOGY AND ONCOLOGY

PROCEDURES DVD AND MANUAL

Kenneth D. Hatch, MD

Professor of Obstetrics and Gynecology
University of Arizona
Tucson, Arizona

Wolters Kluwer | Lippincott Williams & Wilkins
Health
Philadelphia · Baltimore · New York · London
Buenos Aires · Hong Kong · Sydney · Tokyo

Acquisitions Editor: Sonya Seigafuse
Managing Editor: Ryan Shaw
Project Manager: Jennifer Harper
Manufacturing Coordinator: Kathleen Brown
Marketing Manager: Kimberly Schonberger
Design Coordinator: Terry Mallon
Production Services: Aptara, Inc.

530 Walnut Street
Philadelphia, PA 19106 USA
LWW.com

Printed in India.

Library of Congress Cataloging-in-Publication Data

Hatch, Kenneth D.
   Laparoscopy for gynecology and oncology :   procedures DVD and manual / Kenneth D. Hatch.
      p. ; cm.
   Includes bibliographical references and index.
   ISBN-13: 978-0-7817-7033-0
   ISBN-10: 0-7817-7033-5
   1. Generative organs, Female—Endoscopic surgery.   2. Generative organs, Female—Cancer—Endoscopic surgery.   3. Laparoscopic surgery.   I. Title.
   [DNLM: 1. Genital Neoplasms, Female—diagnosis.   2. Laparoscopy—methods.
3. Diagnostic Techniques, Obstetrical and Gynecological. WP 141 H361L 2008]
   RG104.7.H38 2008
   618.1′059—dc22

                                              2007019940

10 9 8 7 6 5 4 3 2 1

This book is dedicated to my wife, Rhea, who has persevered with me and to the hundreds of students, residents, fellows, and physicians who have taught me how to be a teacher.

Preface

Laparoscopy has become the preferred approach to gynecologic surgery since the 1970s. Improved imaging equipment and better surgical tools adapted to the minimally invasive approach have allowed more complicated operations to be performed through the laparoscope. Surgical training for basic laparoscopic skills is available in all the training programs. The more advanced procedures for endometriosis and cancer are less well taught as the number of patients available to the trainee is decreasing.

The ability to see a surgical procedure on video before performing it on a patient improves the trainee surgeon's understanding of the operation and accelerates learning. This surgical manual and video DVD are designed to improve the understanding and accelerate the learning of advanced laparoscopic surgery.

It is a compilation of 16 years of experience in performing and teaching laparoscopic surgery. There have been hundreds of videos collected as better imaging has given the trainee a better view of the anatomy. The use of demonstration and teaching videos has been the most important step in improving the laparoscopic skills of the residents in our program. By viewing the videos, one case becomes many as the resident sees the surgery as often as she or he wishes. My hope for this manual and DVD video is that it will be used by all who wish to improve their skills in laparoscopic surgery.

Contents

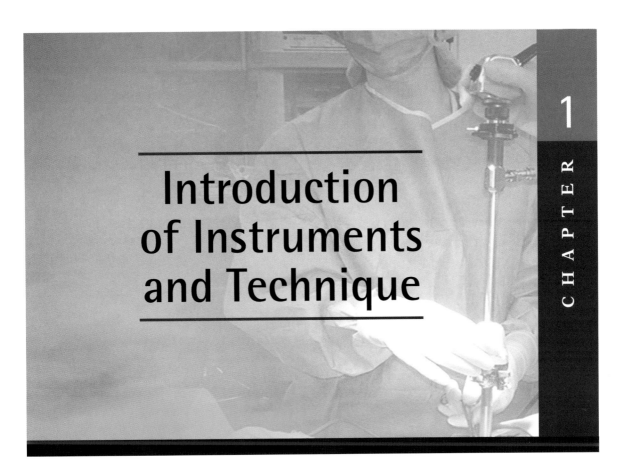

Introduction of Instruments and Technique

The successful performance of laparoscopic surgery is highly dependent upon the equipment. The most important piece of equipment is the video camera. Originally, the cameras were one chip, meaning that the chip processed red, blue, and green colors onto one chip. This resulted in the picture becoming too dark when the field was stained red with blood. In addition to being dark, the detail between tissue planes was diminished so that the perception of depth was absent. The modern camera is a three chip camera with separate chips to detect red, blue, and green. When blood stains the operating field with these cameras, the picture maintains the light and depth of field to a much better degree.

The entry into the abdomen is by trocars inserted through cannulas. The abdomen is most often accessed through the umbilicus. The primary trocar and cannula are inserted through an incision made in the umbilicus. Prior insufflation with a Verres needle to 15 mm Hg pressure CO_2 is recommended when the patient is obese. Direct puncture with a cutting primary cannula can be used in patients who are normal weight and who have not had previous midline abdominal incisions.

FIGURE 1

A primary cannula with a retractable cutting blade, which retracts after the trocar has passed through the fascia and peritoneum, is most often used (Fig. 1-1). This decreases the incidence of vascular injuries to the aorta.

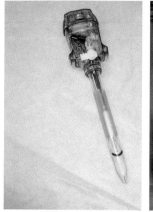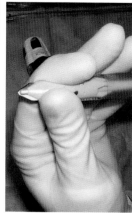

Figure 1-1. Retractable blade cutting trocar.

FIGURE 2

The other type of primary cannula is a plastic tipped tissue separating trocar through which the laparoscope is inserted (Fig. 1-2). The operator can watch the trocar pass through the subcutaneous fat, fascia, preperitoneal fat, and peritoneum as the trocar is turned clockwise. This requires prior insufflation of the abdomen with the Verres needle. This trocar separates the fascia rather than cutting it, and the incidence of vascular injury, as well as port-site hernias, is decreased.

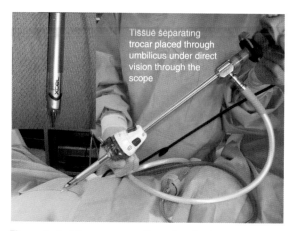

Figure 1-2. Tissue separating plastic tip trocar.

FIGURE 3

The secondary trocars and cannula are placed on the abdomen at the sites demonstrated in Figure 1-3. The lateral port should be lateral to the superficial and deep inferior epigastric arteries; this is lateral to the rectus abdominis muscle. The suprapubic port should be 3 cm above the symphysis to avoid puncture of the bladder. All the cannulas should have a ribbed surface so that the cannulas will not pull out when the operating instruments are placed in and out of the abdomen.

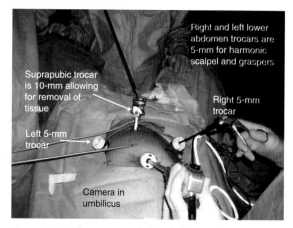

Figure 1-3. Placement of the abdominal trocars.

FIGURE 4

The graspers are generally reusable. For dissection of the lymph nodes, the jaws should be atraumatic and have a width of 4 mm and length of 1.5 cm. This allows the lymph nodes to be grasped and pulled through the 10 mm port with less tearing. For grasping sutures, a hemostat shaped jaw is useful (Fig. 1-4).

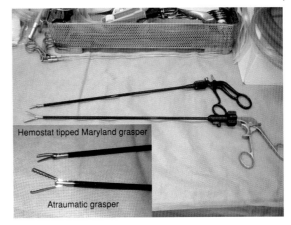

Figure 1-4. Graspers.

FIGURE 5

There have been a variety of instruments and energy used to dissect the lymph nodes, seal the vessels, and cut the vessels. Monopolar cautery transmitted through the laparoscopic scissors was the first method used in our training program (Fig. 1-5). It was able to seal small vessels with an electric current set at 35 watts of power. It would seal and separate the lymph from the vessels quickly. The disadvantage was that heat is generated, which could cause injury. This lead to some postoperative complications of ureterovaginal and vesicovaginal fistula. It required very accurate control of the instrument tip when dissecting around vessels, ureter, and bowel. This level of skill required a number of cases and was a major deterrent to surgeons adopting laparoscopic surgery.

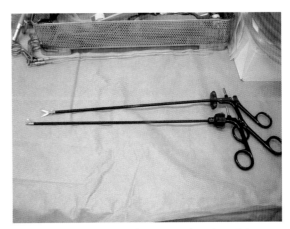

Figure 1-5. Scissors with monopolar electricity.

FIGURE 6

Bipolar electricity has been the most commonly used modality in general gynecology to seal the blood vessels (Fig. 1-6). Its mechanism of action is to desiccate the tissue in the grasping instrument. This requires generation of a large amount of heat. The lateral spread of heat injury is 3 to 5 mm beyond the visible charred area. This also caused postoperative complications of fistula formation. Following desiccation, another instrument was required to cut the desiccated area until the bipolar cutting devices were introduced.

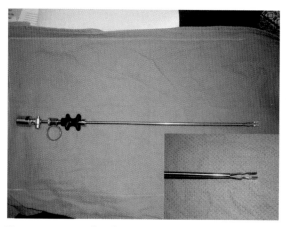

Figure 1-6. Bipolar desiccating instrument.

FIGURE 7

The bipolar cutting instruments were an improvement over the simple grasping instruments. After desiccating the tissue with bipolar current, a knife blade built into the instrument was passed down the center of the jaws to divide the tissue (Fig. 1-7).

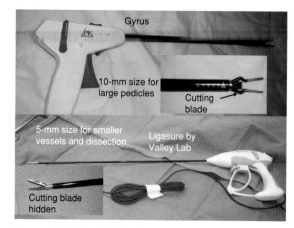

Figure 1-7. Bladed bipolar cutting instruments.

FIGURE 8

It allowed the operator to cut the tissue without introducing another instrument. However, the problem of heat injury around the vessels and ureter still existed. A newer generation of bipolar instruments is now available. The tissue is sealed and divided by the electrical current with only 1 mm of lateral thermal injury (Fig. 1-8).

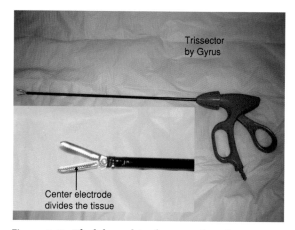

Figure 1-8. Bladeless bipolar cutting instrument 5-mm size.

FIGURE 9

The harmonic scalpel was introduced into our training program to address the above concerns about postoperative complications (Fig. 1-9). It utilizes a rapidly vibrating blade to dissect, seal, and cut. It seals vessels up to 5 mm in diameter at a low temperature not exceeding 100°C. This makes it safe to use around blood vessels, ureter, and bowel. It is ideal for the gynecologic oncology procedure which requires precise dissection around blood vessels, ureter, and bowel with minimal risk of injury. Its ability to seal and cut blood vessels without heat energy is an advantage over electricity. It speeds the operation because the same instrument can be used for dissection, sealing, and cutting. Since the harmonic scalpel was introduced into the program, there has not been a ureterovaginal or vesicovaginal fistula in over 200 cases. The safety of this instrument will encourage the beginning surgeon to adopt laparoscopic surgery into their practice.

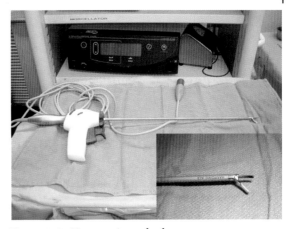

Figure 1-9. Harmonic scalpel.

The surgeon is encouraged to record all of the surgical procedures. Reviewing the videos soon after the surgery allows you to analyze your technique. The ideal recording device is the DVD writer. It allows for up to 2.5 hours of video collection. It is easy to edit digital images with software that is available. Editing the video into segments suitable for teaching also improves the skill of the surgeon. If the surgeon is attempting to show an audience how to do a procedure, he will learn the exposure techniques and camera positioning that improves the viewer's learning.

Now, let's begin learning laparoscopic techniques for gynecologic surgery.

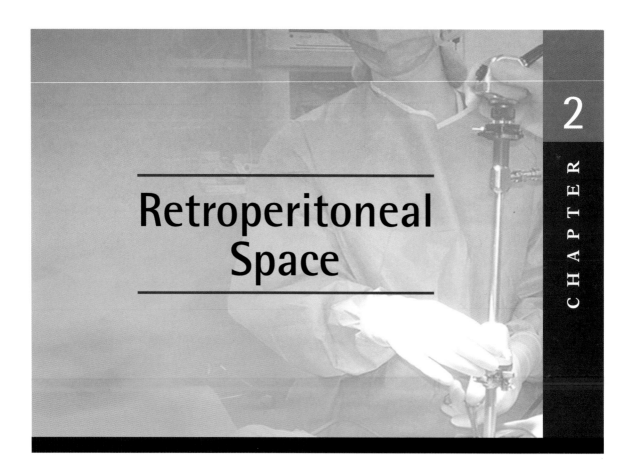

Retroperitoneal Space

To perform advanced gynecologic surgery, the surgeon must know the anatomy of the retroperitoneal space. Many disease processes involve the pelvic peritoneum, uterosacral ligaments, rectosigmoid, or ovarian pedicles, which require the surgeon to enter the retroperitoneal space to identify the ureters and blood vessels and to keep them out of harms way. Badly distorted anatomy of the anterior and posterior cul-de-sac may necessitate mobilization of the rectosigmoid and bladder. Interligamentous fibroids require knowledge of the blood supply in the retroperitoneal space. The surgical treatment and staging of gynecologic malignancies require that the lymph nodes be dissected.

The Ureter

Ureteral injuries occur from 0.5% to 2.5% of women undergoing gynecologic surgery (1). The most common predisposing condition is previous pelvic surgery (2,3). The usual sites of injury are at the pelvic rim close to the ovarian vessels, at the level of the uterine artery, and lateral to the vaginal cuff. Neither preoperative excretory urograms nor placement of ureteral catheters preoperatively have been found to be effective in preventing complications (2,4–6). The blood supply of the ureter comes from plexus of vessels, which forms a network along the length of the ureter. This plexus is fed by arteries from the renal pelvis, common iliac, internal iliac, uterine artery, and the base of the bladder. Complete mobilization of the ureter away from its peritoneal attachments and these lateral blood supply sources can be accomplished as long as the vascular plexus is not disrupted by cautery, crushing, or tearing. A clean transection can be reanastomosed or reimplanted with the expectation of normal healing. Innervation of the ureter is from the inferior mesenteric plexus superiorly and the inferior hypogastric plexus in the pelvis. The ureter will continue to peristalsis even if it is completely divided or ligated.

Pelvic Blood Vessels

Knowledge of the lateral blood vessels is important when the surgeon is faced with a large endometrioma or cancer. Because the pathology is usually deep in the pelvis, it is important to identify the vascular anatomy of the pelvis starting at the pelvic brim where the common iliac bifurcates into the external and internal iliacs. There is a safe dissection plane medial to the internal iliac all the way to the uterine artery. This exposes the perirectal space that can be opened without risk of major bleeding. The obliterated umbilical vessel is the other marker just distal to the uterine artery. It can be placed on traction so the uterine artery can be isolated. The middle and superior vesical arteries are generally not dissected because they are adjacent to the bladder, and the surgery takes place medial to them in the prevesical fascial space. The obturator artery will only be exposed if the surgeon is dissecting the obturator lymph nodes for a cancer operation. Ligation of the hypogastric artery is rarely performed today, as embolization by interventional radiology is the standard of care for the postoperative and postpartum bleeding patient. If acute bleeding from the hypogastric artery occurs during laparoscopic surgery, immediate pressure followed by a 10-mm hemoclip may control the bleeding. This is only possible if the ureter has been previously dissected out of harms way. If bleeding continues, it is best to convert to open surgery with appropriate consultation. While performing the laparotomy, pressure should be placed on the artery with a grasper. When it becomes necessary, the hypogastric artery can be isolated and tied using the right-angle clamp to pass the tie. The superior gluteal artery branches so close to the bifurcation of the common iliac that it is not visualized. The inferior gluteal artery is the largest distal branch which might be visualized during the ligation; however, it is not necessary to identify it.

The Pelvic Nerves

The genitofemoral nerve runs along the medial aspect of the body of the psoas muscle. It is sometimes injured by the self-retaining retractors placed at the time of laparotomy, which leads to numbness and burning of the skin of the anterior thigh. The obturator nerve is in the obturator space and usually far lateral to the usual dissection. Metastatic cancer to the obturator lymph nodes may entrap it or it may be injured during a node dissection. Loss of internal rotation of the anterior thigh results from the injury. The sciatic nerve is only seen during exenterative surgery. Pressure on the lateral pelvis by advanced pelvic tumors can lead to sciatic pain and motor weakness, which leads to loss of motor function to the lower leg, most commonly leading to foot drop.

The hypogastric plexus of nerves are sometimes damaged during surgery for endometriosis or for malignancy. The superior hypogastric plexus can be identified between the two common iliac arteries at the sacral promontory. The left common iliac vein runs underneath it. The right and left hypogastric nerves leave the hypogastric plexus and descend into the pelvis parallel to the ureter and 2 cm medial. It passes dorsal to the ureter as it goes through the cardinal ligament. This plexus then supplies autonomic enervation of the bladder, rectum, uterus, and ureter. Complete disruption of the hypogastric nerve will lead to a hypertonic, noncontractile bladder and the necessity to self-cath to eliminate urine. Preservation of this nerve during performance of a radical hysterectomy or in resecting endometriosis should be a high priority. The laparoscopic uterosacral nerve ablation procedures divide the uterosacral ligament medial and caudad to the ureter and do not disrupt the main hypogastric nerve. Only the branches medial to the uterus are affected. Uterosacral nerve ablation has been reported to be successful in approximately 44% of the women who have dysmenorrhea without visible endometriosis and in approximately 62% of women who have visible endometriosis (7,8). There is controversy concerning the efficacy of this procedure. Removal of the superior hypogastric plexus (presacral neurectomy) has not been shown to be more effective in controlling pelvic pain than conservative surgery that only destroys endometrial implants. Presacral neurectomy is no longer advised (9).

The operative technique to expose the retroperitoneal anatomy of the pelvis

STEP 1

The patient is placed in the low lithotomy position with adjustable stirrups. The arms are tucked to each side and an oropharyngeal tube is placed (Fig. 2-1).

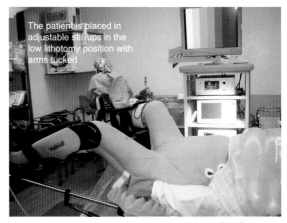

Figure 2-1. Patient position.

STEP 2

The surgeon stands on the patient's right side to dissect the left pelvis. The camera is placed in the umbilical port and held in the assistant's right hand. The assistant's left hand holds a grasper in the left lower abdominal port. The surgeon places medial traction on the left round ligament with the grasper in the suprapubic port. The harmonic scalpel seals and divides the left round ligament (Fig. 2-2).

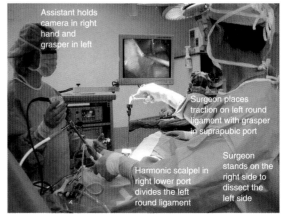

Figure 2-2. Position of the surgeon and assistant.

STEP 3

The round ligament is the first anatomic structure that should be identified to expose the retroperitoneal space. It should be opened at the pelvic sidewall, just medial to the external iliac vessels. The round ligament crosses the umbilical ligament at this point and can be exposed after transecting the round ligament (Fig. 2-3).

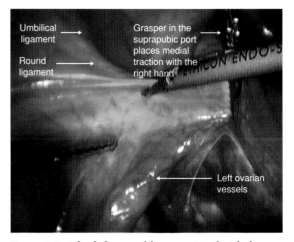

Figure 2-3. The left round ligament is divided.

STEP 4

The divided round ligament is retracted ventrally and medially to place the ovarian vessels under traction. The peritoneum lateral to the ovarian vessels is divided up to the pelvic brim (Fig. 2-4).

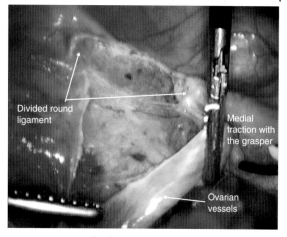

Figure 2-4. Divide the peritoneum lateral to the left ovarian vessels.

STEP 5

The umbilical ligament is exposed in the broad ligament dorsal to the opened round ligament (Fig. 2-5).

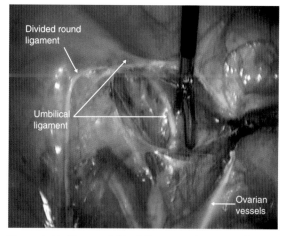

Figure 2-5. The umbilical ligament is exposed.

STEP 6

Medial traction of the peritoneum around the ovarian vessels at the pelvic brim will expose the ureter over the iliac vessels at their bifurcation into external and internal branches (Fig. 2-6).

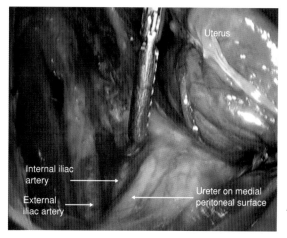

Figure 2-6. The left ureter is exposed at the pelvic brim.

STEP 7

The ureter comes off medial with the fold of peritoneum. Once the space is developed, the laparoscopic probe can be introduced along the medial side of the internal iliac artery and ventral to the curve of the sacrum. This will open the pararectal space (Fig. 2-7).

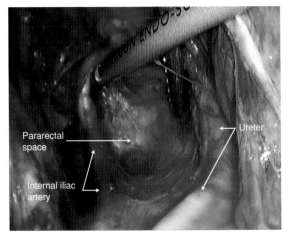

Figure 2-7. The pararectal space is developed.

STEP 8

The umbilical ligament was the umbilical artery in fetal life and courses along the edge of the bladder to the anterior abdominal wall up to the umbilicus. It is a useful structure to guide one into the perivesical space. The umbilical ligament is dissected away from the parauterine tissue. This exposes the perivesical space (Fig. 2-8).

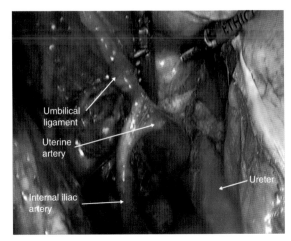

Figure 2-8. The paravesical space medial to the umbilical ligament is opened.

STEP 9

The uterine artery is isolated. It can be divided at its origin from the internal iliac artery for resection of cancer or endometriosis (Fig. 2-9).

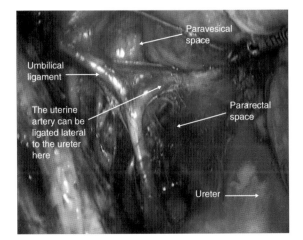

Figure 2-9. The left uterine artery is isolated at its origin from the internal iliac artery.

Endometriosis

Endometriosis is one of the most common reasons for accessing the retroperitoneal space. Complete surgical removal of the endometriomas and the peritoneal implants is considered an important step to eliminate the pain associated with it. Frequently, the peritoneum between the ovarian vessels and the uterosacral ligaments (ovarian fossa) is thickened and retracted within the endometriosis implants. This alters the pelvic anatomy and puts the ureter at risk for injury. Definitive surgical treatment for endometriosis includes removal of this diseased peritoneum. The ureter will need to be identified and dissected off the peritoneum down to the uterine artery. The cul-de-sac of Douglas is another site of endometrial implants. The fundus of the uterus is often adhesed to the rectosigmoid reflection and even the sigmoid colon. Nodules of endometriosis may be infiltrating the uterosacral ligaments and extending down into the rectovaginal space. These implants may be managed by isolating the ureter down to the point that it passes under the uterine artery. The uterine artery is often transected lateral to the mass, which enables the surgeon to remove all of the uterosacral implants. As the dissection proceeds medially, the perirectal fatty plane is used to remove the implants between the uterosacral and rectum. In the midline, implants that are below the rectosigmoid peritoneal reflexion can be removed with care not to injure the rectum. Implants above the peritoneal reflexion are often attached to the sigmoid tinea coli and cannot be removed without taking a portion of the bowel. Thus, patients that have extensive endometriosis should have a bowel prep with two 10 oz. bottles of magnesium citrate the day before surgery so that the bowel resection can be preformed safely. If bowel resection does become necessary, a general surgeon or gynecologic oncologist should be consulted. A history of painful defecation or a physical finding of nodules in the cul-de-sac with dimpling of the rectum should prompt a preoperative consultation with a specialist with skills in bowel resection.

Resection of endometriosis using the retroperitoneal space

STEP 1

Transect the round ligament where it crosses the umbilical ligament (Fig. 2-10). The surgeon is on the patient's right side to operate in the left pelvis.

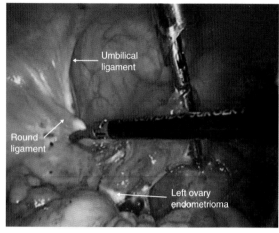

Figure 2-10. Resection of endometriosis begins with dividing the round ligament at the umbilical ligament.

STEP 2

Incise the peritoneum lateral to the ovarian vessels. Put medial traction with the grasper in the suprapubic port (Fig. 2-11).

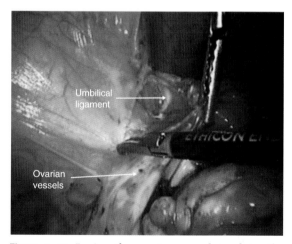

Figure 2-11. Incise the peritoneum lateral to the ovarian vessels.

STEP 3

Expose the ureter at the pelvic brim (Figs. 2-12 and 2-13). The assistant is retracting the sigmoid colon with the left mid-abdomen grasper.

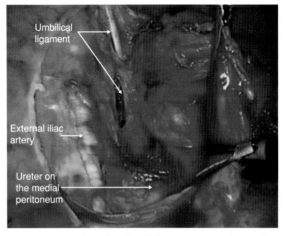

Figure 2-12. Identify the left ureter at the pelvic brim.

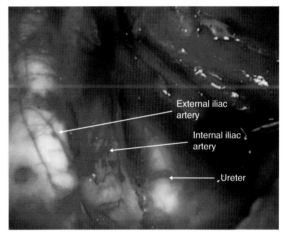

Figure 2-13. Close-up of the relationship of ureter to the iliac vessels.

STEP 4

Develop the pararectal and paravesical space (Fig. 2-14).

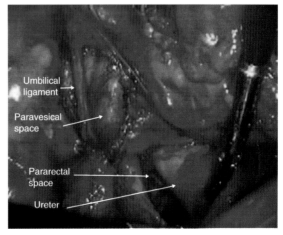

Figure 2-14. Open the pararectal and paravesical spaces.

STEP 5

Isolate the uterine artery and divide it lateral to the ureter (Fig. 2-15).

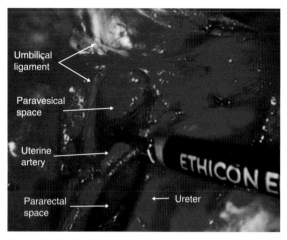

Figure 2-15. Isolate the uterine artery and transect lateral to the ureter.

STEP 6

Dissect the ureter off the peritoneum to remove all of the endometriosis (Fig. 2-16). The uterine artery is retracted ventrally to bring it over the ureter.

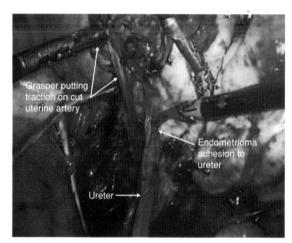

Figure 2-16. Dissect the left ureter from the endometriosis.

STEP 7

Dissect the right ureter off the endometrioma (Fig. 2-17). The dissection should be medial to the ureter. Rarely is resection of the ureter necessary.

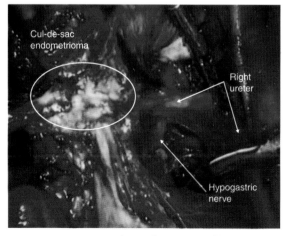

Figure 2-17. Dissect the right ureter off the cul-de-sac endometriosis.

STEP 8

Dissect the sigmoid colon away from the cul-de-sac endometrioma (Fig. 2-18). Dissection in the yellow fat plane is safe. The heat of the harmonic scalpel is <100°C.

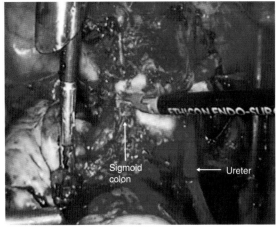

Figure 2-18. Dissect the sigmoid away from the cul-de-sac endometriosis.

STEP 9

Complete the rectovaginal space dissection so that the operation can go to the vaginal side (Fig. 2-19). When the rectovaginal fat plane is reached and the ureters are lateral, it is easier to finish vaginally.

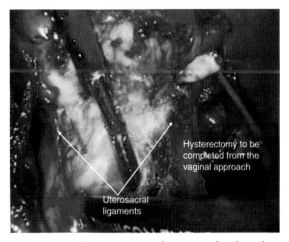

Figure 2-19. The rectovaginal space is developed.

STEP 10

The appearance of the right and left pelvis after completion of the hysterectomy from vaginal route (Figs. 2-20 and 2-21).

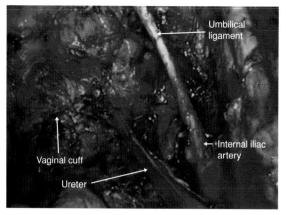

Figure 2-20. The postoperative appearance of the right pelvis.

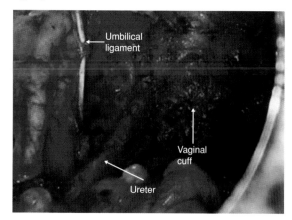

Figure 2-21. The postoperative appearance of the left pelvis.

References

1. American College of Obstetricians and Gynecologists. *Lower Urinary Tract Operative Injuries* (ACOG Educational Bulletin No. 238). Washington, DC: American College of Obstetricians and Gynecologists. 1985;1.

2. Daly JW, Higgins KA. Injury to the ureter during gynecologic surgical procedures. *Surg Gynecol Obstet.* 1988;167:19–22.

3. Selzman AA, Spirnak JP. Iatrogenic ureteral injuries: a 20-year experience in treating 165 injuries. *J Urol.* 1996;155:878–881.

4. Symmonds RE. Ureteral injuries associated with gynecologic surgery: prevention and management. *Clin Obstet Gynecol.* 1976;19:623–644.

5. Higgins CC. Ureteral injuries during surgery: a review of 87 cases. *J Amer Med Assoc.* 1967;199:82–88.

6. Fry DE, Milholen L, Harbrecht PJ. Iatrogenic ureteral injury. Options in management. *Arch Surg.* 1983;118:454–457.

7. Lichten EM, Bombard J. Surgical treatment of primary dysmenorrhea with laparoscopic uterine nerve ablation. *J Reprod Med.* 1987;32:37–41.

8. Sutton CJG, Ewen SP, Whitelaw N, et al. Prospective, randomized, double-blind, controlled trial of laser laparoscopy in the treatment of pelvic pain associated with minimal, mild, and moderate endometriosis. *Fertil Steril.* 1994;62:696.

9. Candiani GB, Fedele L, Vercellini P, et al. Presacral neurectomy for the treatment of pelvic pain associated with endometriosis: a controlled study. *Amer J Obstet Gynecol.* 1992;167:100–103.

Development of Laparoscopic Surgery for Gynecologic Oncology

aparoscopy has been widely accepted in gynecology since the mid-1960s. Initially it was performed by a single surgeon looking through a single eyepiece, which limited the surgery to simple operations such as tubal ligations. Today, laparoscopy is performed with three-chip cameras processing red, green, and blue signals transmitted to video monitors that can be viewed by all of the operating and nursing team. It allows the surgeon, as well as the assistants, full view of the operation and thus the ability to perform extensive operations similar to open surgery. The principles of open surgery apply to laparoscopic surgery.

- The operative field must be adequately exposed.
- The anatomy must be identified.
- The tissue to be removed must be accessible.
- The surgeon must have the knowledge and skill to perform the operation.

Video laparoscopy was rapidly adapted to simple gynecologic procedures such as adnexal mass removal, laparoscopically assisted vaginal hysterectomy, adhesiolysis, and removal of endometriosis. It was not assimilated into gynecologic oncology because a technique for removal of pelvic and para-aortic lymph nodes did not exist.

The performance of a pelvic and para-aortic lymphadenectomy, either a partial lymphadenectomy (lymph node sampling) or complete lymphadenectomy, is the key procedure for the staging of gynecologic malignancies.

Laparoscopic Pelvic and Para–aortic Lymphadenectomy

In 1989, French surgeons, Dargent and Salvat (1), used the laparoscope to perform limited pelvic lymphadenectomy in women with cervical cancer. This was not widely accepted because of its limited access to the pelvic lymph nodes and the inability to evaluate the lymph nodes in the common iliac and para-aortic chains. In 1991, Childers and Surwit (2) described pelvic and para-aortic lymphadenectomy performed in conjunction with a laparoscopically assisted vaginal hysterectomy and bilateral salpingo-oophorectomy in two women with endometrial cancer. In 1992, Nezhat et al. (3) published a case of laparoscopic radical hysterectomy and pelvic and para-aortic lymphadenectomy, although the dissection with only 2 cm above the aortic bifurcation yielded an inadequate evaluation. These early publications were limited case reports that gave no information on morbidity, mortality, or complications.

Querleu et al. (4) performed transperitoneal laparoscopic pelvic lymphadenectomy in 39 patients with cervical cancer. Five patients had metastatic lymph nodes and were treated with radiation therapy. Thirty-two patients underwent abdominal radical hysterectomy and evaluation of the completeness of the laparoscopic lymphadenectomy. The sensitivity for node positivity by laparoscopy was 100%. However, the number of additional lymph nodes found at laparotomy was not stated.

Childers et al. (5) reported 59 patients with endometrial cancer who were staged laparoscopically, followed by vaginal hysterectomy and bilateral salpingo-oophorectomy. Six patients were found to have intraperitoneal disease and did not receive a lymphadenectomy. Twenty-two patients had grade 1 disease with less than one-half myometrial invasion and did not have a lymphadenectomy. Thirty-one patients should have had lymph node staging, but obesity precluded it in two patients, giving a feasibility rate of 93%. Three major and three minor complications were reported. The surgical complications were experienced early in the series and led to alternative techniques as the series progressed. The average hospital stay was 2.9 days, but information pertaining to the operative time, lymph node counts, and cost analysis was not available.

These early series emphasized pelvic lymphadenectomy, but it remained necessary to do para-aortic lymphadenectomy for laparoscopy to be fully accepted as a technique to stage all gynecologic malignancies. Childers et al. (6) reported both pelvic and para-aortic lymphadenectomy in 16 of 18 patients being treated for cervical cancer. Two patients did not have para-aortic lymphadenectomies because of obesity. Para-aortic lymphadenectomies were performed from the right side of the aorta and included the entire chain from the duodenum to the bifurcation. Eight of the 18 patients underwent laparoscopic staging before planned radical hysterectomy. Three of the eight patients had positive pelvic lymph nodes at the time of laparoscopy and were treated with radiation therapy. The remaining five patients had radical hysterectomies immediately after the laparoscopic lymphadenectomy. The average number of lymph nodes removed at laparoscopy was 31, with an average of three additional lymph nodes being found at laparotomy. There were no additional positive pelvic or para-aortic lymph nodes found on laparotomy. For patients having only laparoscopy, the average hospital stay was 1.5 days, with a blood loss 50 mL, and operative time of 75 to 175 minutes.

Fowler et al. (7) performed laparoscopic lymphadenectomies on 12 patients with cervical cancer. Two of those had right-sided para-aortic lymphadenectomy performed to the level of the inferior mesenteric artery. All patients underwent laparotomy after the laparoscopic dissection to evaluate the completeness of the lymphadenectomy; an average of 23 lymph nodes were removed by laparoscopy, and an additional seven lymph nodes were removed by laparotomy. Two patients had positive lymph nodes, and both of these were identified by laparoscopy. The "learning curve" was documented by showing an increase in the percentage of lymph nodes removed by laparoscopy from 63% in the first six patients to 85% in the second six patients. It is important to note that all of the positive lymph nodes were identified and removed using the laparoscope. All complications were related to the hysterectomy and included transfusion in three patients and cellulitis in one patient. Laparoscopy significantly added to the combined operative time, which averaged 373 minutes. Querleu et al. (4), Childers et al. (5,6), and Fowler et al. (7) all used laparotomy to confirm the accuracy of lymphadenectomy, and in each report, all positive lymph nodes were identified.

Childers et al. (8) summarized the Arizona experience in para-aortic lymphadenectomy through 1993 with a report of 61 women with cervical, endometrial, or ovarian cancer. In three patients (5%), obesity prevented the completion of the surgery, and in one patient (0.8%), adhesions were responsible for failure. Lymph node counts were available in 23 patients: For the right-sided dissection, there was an average lymph node count of three. For the six patients who underwent a bilateral para-aortic lymphadenectomy, operative time ranged from 25 to

70 minutes, and the average hospital stay for the 33 patients with laparoscopic lymphadenectomy was only 1.3 days. There was one vena caval injury that required transfusion and laparotomy, which is a comparable rate to open surgery.

In 1994, Querleu and LeBlanc (9) described a laparoscopic infrarenal para-aortic lymphadenectomy for staging of cancer of the ovary or fallopian tube in nine patients. An average of nine nodes were removed, with an operative time of 111 minutes, an average postoperative stay of 2.8 days, and a blood loss <300 mL in all patients. None of the lymph nodes were positive.

In 1995, Spirtos et al. (10) reported 40 patients with bilateral partial para-aortic lymphadenectomy (sampling). Five laparotomies were performed: Two to remove unsuspected metastases, two for control of hemorrhage, and one because of equipment failure. In two patients, the left-sided dissection was judged to be inadequate, which is an overall failure rate of 12.5%. An average of eight para-aortic lymph nodes were removed: Four from the right side and four from the left side. Most of the patients also underwent a pelvic lymphadenectomy and hysterectomy; the mean operative time was 193 minutes, and the average hospital stay was 2.9 days.

Possover et al. (11) reported the accuracy of laparoscopic assessment of the pelvic and para-aortic lymph nodes. Eighty-four patients with cervical cancer underwent laparoscopic lymphadenectomy. The surgeon classified the lymph nodes as positive or negative by visualization. The sensitivity and specificity of visualization was 92.3%. When frozen-section analysis was combined with laparoscopic assessment, 100% of the positive lymph nodes were identified. In 13 of the 84 patients, the treatment plan was altered during surgery based on these findings.

Possover et al. (12) analyzed videotapes of 112 para-aortic lymphadenectomies and detailed the ventral tributaries of the infrarenal vena cava. They divided the vena cava into three levels based on the distribution of venous tributaries. This is a significant contribution to anatomic knowledge and is an important guide for beginning laparoscopic surgeons.

Multiple recent studies continue to report the adequacy and safety of laparoscopic pelvic and para-aortic node dissections in gynecologic cancer (13–16). These studies demonstrate the ability of laparoscopic surgeons to perform pelvic and para-aortic lymphadenectomy. The American Medical Association Physicians Current Procedure Terminology (CPT 2004) lists a total of four laparoscopic lymph node dissection procedures, including total pelvic lymphadenectomy and para-aortic lymph node sampling. Since then, laparoscopic surgery has been used by more oncologic surgeons and has been applied to nearly every disease site in gynecologic oncology.

Technique

Lymphadenectomy

Preoperative Preparation

Patient preparation begins with a clear liquid diet the day before the surgical procedure. Evacuation of the bowel may be accomplished with magnesium citrate or Go-Lytely. It is important for the bowel to be collapsed during the laparoscopic lymphadenectomy so that proper exposure can be obtained. This is particularly important if the patient is somewhat obese and para-aortic lymphadenectomy is planned.

Operative Approach

The recommended technique of laparoscopy is as follows:

STEP 1

The patient is positioned in a dorsal lithotomy position with legs in stirrups that support the legs and decrease the tension on the femoral and peroneal nerves (Fig. 3-1). It is helpful to have adjustable stirrups that allow for conversion from the low lithotomy to a leg-flexed position for vaginal surgery. The arms are tucked at each side, an endotracheal tube is positioned, and a Foley catheter is placed in the bladder.

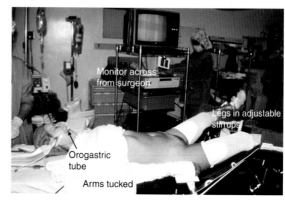

Figure 3-1. Patient position.

STEP 2

The first trocar is inserted into the umbilicus if the patient does not have a midline incision. If there is a midline incision, then a left upper quadrant insufflation and 5-mm trocar are used. The left upper quadrant approach for patients with previous midline incisions allows the laparoscope to be placed away from possible adhesions that can then be dissected from the umbilicus before placing the 10-mm trocar.

STEP 3

Additional 5-mm trocars are placed in the right and left lower quadrants and in the suprapubic site. Typically, a 10-mm trocar is placed in the suprapubic site to remove lymph nodes. Also, the laparoscope can be placed in that port to help with packing the bowel or in dissecting adhesions from around the umbilical port (Fig. 3-2).

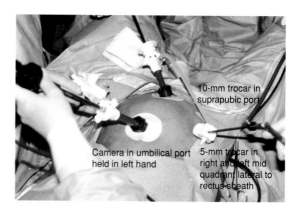

Figure 3-2. Location of trocars.

STEP 4

The bowel should be carefully packed into the upper abdomen so that adequate exposure of the para-aortic area and pelvis can be obtained. Sponges or minilaparotomy packs can be placed around loops of bowel to aid in exposure and to blot small amounts of blood. The principles of laparoscopic surgery are the same as those of laparotomy. There must be adequate exposure, identification of the anatomy, and removal of the appropriate tissue.

STEP 5

The lymphadenectomies are best performed by the surgeon on the side opposite the side of dissection (i.e., the surgeon on the patient's right side dissects the left pelvic lymph nodes). The peritoneal incisions are left open and drains are not placed.

STEP 6

The para-aortic lymphadenectomy is usually performed first. Both the right- and left-sided aortic lymph nodes are sampled. The peritoneum is incised between the sigmoid mesentery and the mesentery of the cecum.

STEP 7

The surgeon is on the patient's left side to perform the right para-aortic node dissection (Fig. 3-3). The left hand holds a grasper that is in the suprapubic port. The right hand holds the dissecting instrument (harmonic scalpel) (Fig. 3-4).

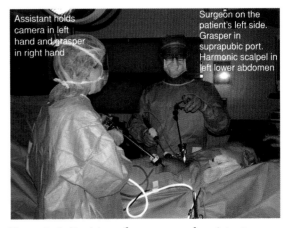

Figure 3-3. Position of surgeon and assistant.

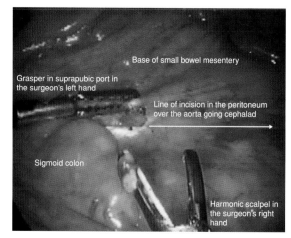

Figure 3-4. Opening the peritoneum over the para-aortic nodes.

STEP 8

The landmarks are usually the reflection of the duodenum and inferior mesenteric vessel superiorly and the psoas muscles laterally. The lymph node chain is isolated and dissection is carried out. Monopolar surgery, bipolar surgery, harmonic scalpel, and the argon beam coagulator have all been used successfully (Fig. 3-5).

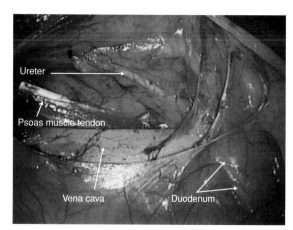

Figure 3-5. The peritoneum is open to the duodenum.

STEP 9

The ureter must be identified and placed on traction by the assistant to keep it out of the operative field. The grasper places ventral traction on the node bundle and the harmonic scalpel divides the tissue vertically along the aorta up to the duodenum (Fig. 3-6). The vena cava is exposed. The perforators can be identified and sealed (Fig. 3-7).

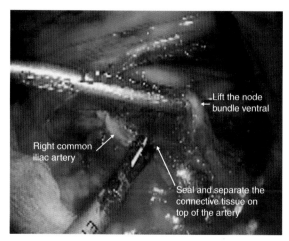

Figure 3-6. Begin the para-aortic dissection on the right common iliac artery.

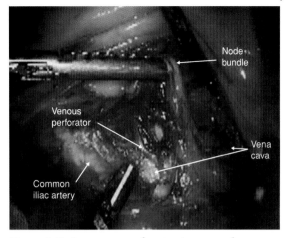

Figure 3-7. A venous perforator is exposed.

STEP 10

The node bundle is transected at the cau-dad end, usually about the mid-common iliac artery (Fig. 3-8). The nodes are then placed on ventral traction while the dissection goes cephalad. At the reflection of the duodenum, the nodes are transected and pulled out the suprapubic port (Figs. 3-9 and 3-10).

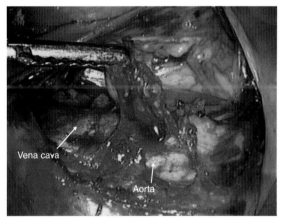

Figure 3-8. The caudad end of the nodes is divided and elevated.

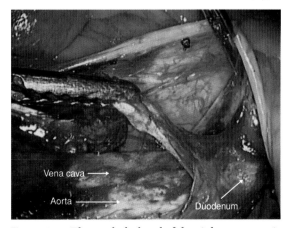

Figure 3-9. The cephalad end of the right para-aortic nodes is exposed.

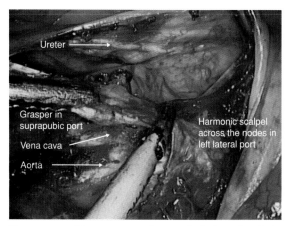

Figure 3-10. Transecting the cephalad end of the right para-aortic nodes.

STEP 11

The left para-aortic nodes are dissected with the surgeon on the patient's right side. The mesentery of the sigmoid is placed on ventral traction and the plane between the mesentery, and the common iliac is developed. The left ureter and the inferior mesenteric artery are identified (Fig. 3-11).

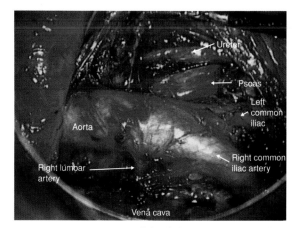

Figure 3-11. Exposure of the left para-aortic nodes.

STEP 12

The lymph nodes on the left side are more lateral and dorsal than on the right (precaval) side. Lifting up the left common iliac artery can mobilize the node bundle dorsally so that it can be picked up with the suprapubic port grasper ventral to the arteries (Fig. 3-12).

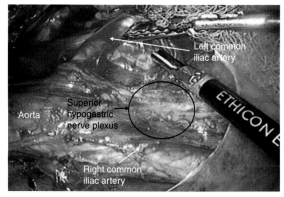

Figure 3-12. Exposing the left common iliac nodes behind the artery.

STEP 13

The node bundle is transected caudad at the mid common iliac artery and placed on ventral traction while the nodes are dissected cephalad to the root of the inferior mesenteric artery (Fig. 3-13). A dissection above the inferior mesenteric artery can be accomplished up to the renal vessels if needed.

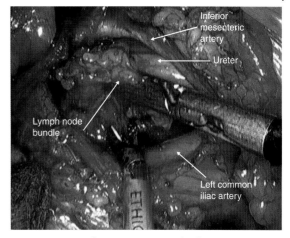

Figure 3-13. Left para-aortic node dissection.

STEP 14

The proximal common iliac lymph nodes are dissected through the retroperitoneal incision made from the para-aortic lymph nodes down to the middle common iliac lymph nodes. The remaining common iliac lymph nodes are dissected through the incision for the pelvic lymphadenectomy (Fig. 3-14).

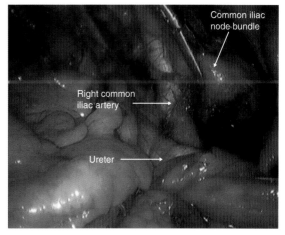

Figure 3-14. Removing the right common iliac nodes through the pelvic excision.

The disease and clinical circumstance determine the extent of the pelvic lymphadenectomy. The technique for each of these will be discussed in the chapter on the disease site.

All port sites 10 mm or larger should have the fascia and peritoneal layers closed to prevent herniation of bowel. Several instruments are available that pass the suture through the skin incision lateral to the port and back up on the opposite side. The skin is closed and a local anesthetic is injected around the port sites to decrease postoperative pain.

References

1. Dargent D, Salvat J. *Envahissenent ganglionnaire pelvien: place de la pelviscopie retroperitoneale.* Paris: Medsi, McGraw-Hill, 1989.
2. Childers J, Surwit E. A combined laparoscopic vaginal approach in the management of stage I endometrial cancer. *Gynecol Oncol.* 1991;45:46–51.
3. Nezhat C, Burrell M, Nezhat F. Laparoscopic radical hysterectomy with para-aortic and pelvic node dissection. *Am J Obstet Gynecol.* 1992;166:864–865.

4. Querleu D, LeBlanc E, Castelain B. Laparoscopic pelvic lymphadenectomy in the staging of early carcinoma of the cervix. *Am J Obstet Gynecol.* 1991;164:579–581.

5. Childers J, Brzechffa P, Hatch K, et al. Laparoscopically assisted surgical staging (LASS) of endometrial cancer. *Gynecol Oncol.* 1992;51:33–38.

6. Childers J, Hatch K, Surwit E. The role of laparoscopic lymphadenectomy in the management of cervical carcinoma. *Gynecol Oncol.* 1992;47:38–43.

7. Fowler J, Carter J, Carlson JW, et al. Lymph node yield from laparoscopic lymphadenectomy in cervical cancer: a comparative study. *Gynecol Oncol.* 1993;51:187–192.

8. Childers J, Hatch K, Tran A-H, et al. Laparoscopic para-aortic lymphadenectomy in gynecologic malignancies. *Obstet Gynecol.* 1993;82:741–747.

9. Querleu D, LeBlanc E. Laparoscopic infrarenal para-aortic lymph node dissection for restaging of carcinoma of the ovary or fallopian tube. *Cancer* 1994;73:1467–1471.

10. Spirtos NM, Schlaerth JB, Spirtos TW, et al. Laparoscopic bilateral pelvic and para-aortic lymph node sampling: an evolving technique. *Am J Obstet Gynecol.* 1995;173:105–111.

11. Possover M, Krause N, Kuhne-Heid R, et al. Value of laparoscopic evaluation of para-aortic and pelvic lymph nodes for treatment of cervical cancer. *Am J Obstet Gynecol.* 1998;178:806–810.

12. Possover M, Plaul K, Krause N, et al. Left-sided laparoscopic para-aortic lymphadenectomy: anatomy of the ventral tributaries of the infrarenal vena cava. *Am J Obstet Gynecol.* 1998;179:1295–1297.

13. Kohler C, Tozzi R, Kelmm P, et al. Laparoscopic para-aortic left-sided transperitoneal infrarenal lymphadenectomy in patients with gynecologic malignancies: technique and results. *Gynecol Oncol.* 2003;91:139–148.

14. Spirtos NM, Eisenkop SM, Schlaerth JB, et al. Laparoscopic radical hysterectomy (type III) with aortic and pelvic lymphadenectomy in patients with stage I cervical cancer surgical morbidity and intermediate follow-up. *Am J Obstet Gynecol.* 2002;187:340–348.

15. Hertel H, Kohler C, Michels W, et al. Laparoscopic-assisted radical vaginal hysterectomy (LARVH): prospective evaluation of 200 patients with cervical cancer. *Gynecol Oncol.* 2003;90:505–511.

16. Gemignani ML, Curtin JP, Zelmanovich J, et al. Laparoscopic-assisted vaginal hysterectomy for endometrial cancer: clinical outcomes and hospital charges. *Gynecol Oncol.* 1999;73:5–11.

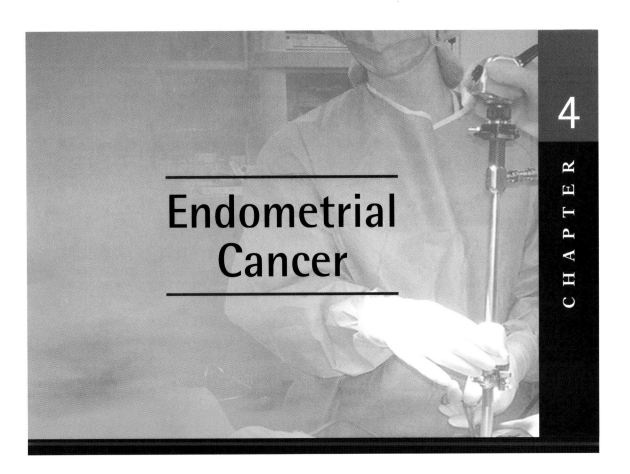

Endometrial Cancer

Most women with endometrial cancer present with disease confined to the uterus. The treatment consists of total hysterectomy, bilateral salpingo-oophorectomy, and surgical staging, which includes peritoneal washings, inspection of the abdomen, and retroperitoneal lymph node sampling. Surgical staging with operative laparoscopy followed by vaginal hysterectomy or laparoscopic total hysterectomy has been proposed as an alternative to laparotomy (1–7).

Childers et al. (8,9) reported two patients in 1992 who underwent laparoscopic staging of the retroperitoneal nodes followed by vaginal hysterectomy and bilateral salpingo-oophorectomy, and presented the first large series in 1993. Laparoscopic staging was successfully performed in 93% of the patients, with obesity noted as a limiting factor. Two patients had complications related to the hysterectomy: One had a transected ureter caused by the endoscopic stapler and one had a cystotomy. The endoscopic stapler is not recommended for use on the cardinal ligaments during a laparoscopically assisted vaginal hysterectomy.

Spirtos et al. (5) reported 13 patients who underwent laparoscopic staging and hysterectomy and compared them with 17 patients who underwent laparotomy. The laparotomy group required significantly longer hospitalization than the laparoscopic group (6.3 vs. 2.4 days, $p < 0.001$), incurred higher overall hospital costs ($19,158 vs. $13,988, $p < 0.05$), and took longer to return to normal activity (5.3 weeks vs. 2.4 weeks, $p < 0.0001$). The patients having laparotomy were significantly obese and had a higher body mass index (30.2 vs. 24.2).

The effect of surgical experience has been demonstrated by Melendez et al. (6). In the first 100 patients with endometrial cancer, the operative time for staging decreased from a mean of 196 minutes for the first 25 patients to 128 minutes for the last 25 patients, and the hospital stay decreased from 3.2 days to 1.8 days. The decrease in operative time and hospital stay, coupled with the diminished use of expensive, disposable instruments, has led to a significant cost savings for laparoscopy and important social benefits for the individual patients.

Table 4–1 Recurrence Rates for Laparoscopic Surgery vs. Laparotomy

		Laparoscopy			Laparotomy	
Reference	No.	Months Follow-up	Recurrence (%)	No.	Months Follow-up	Recurrence (%)
Gemignani (11)	59	18	6%	235	30	7%
El Tabbakh (16)	100	27	7%	86	48	10%
Malur (17)	37	16	3%	33	16	3%
Holub (13)	177	33	6%	44	45	7%
Hatch (18)	111	33	7%	55	33	14%

Recent publications have continued to show a decrease in operative time, hospital stay, and total cost for laparoscopic treatment of endometrial cancer (10–12).

Women with endometrial cancer are often obese with body mass index (BMI) >35 (13). This has been thought to be a limiting factor in using laparoscopy to stage and treat endometrial cancer. As surgical skills have advanced, laparoscopy has been successfully used in these women. Holub et al. (14) has successfully completed staging and hysterectomies in 94.4% of 33 patients with BMI of 30 to 40. Eltabbakh et al. (15) has completed staging in 88% of 42 women with BMIs of 28 to 60. In both studies, the benefits of shorter hospital stay with faster recovery were verified.

Long-term survival has been reported in five papers (Table 4-1). More than 480 patients have been followed for a median of 18 to 34 months, with recurrence rates of 2.5% to 7%. When compared to historical laparotomy controls in these papers, there was no difference in survival.

The concept of sentinel node removal has been studied in endometrial cancer in two pilot studies. Holub et al. (19) injected blue dye either into the subserosal myometrium (13 patients) or the cervix and subserosal myometrium (12 patients). Sentinel nodes were most often found in the cervicosubserosal myometrium (83% vs. 61%). Garguilo (20) used both radioactive isotope injection into the cervix and blue dye in 11 patients. Seventeen sentinel nodes were identified and included all three of the positive nodes found after complete node dissection. Further studies are warranted in endometrial cancer.

Technique

Laparoscopic Assisted Vaginal Hysterectomy Bilateral Salpingoophorectomy and Lymph Node Dissection for Endometrial Cancer

Patients with grade 2 and 3 tumors should have a pelvic and para-aortic node lymph node dissection performed as a part of their staging and treatment. It is recommended that these women have the node dissection done first, followed by the laparoscopic assisted vaginal hysterectomy (LAVH) and bilateral salpingo-oophorectomy (BSO). Women with grade 1 tumors should have a node dissection in the following situations: (i) if the tumor is beyond the inner half of the myometrium, (ii) it extends to the cervix, (iii) it extends to the adnexa, or (iv) it is a more advanced grade. For these patients, an LAVH BSO followed by a frozen section is recommended to determine if the above factors are present before proceeding with the node dissection.

The para-aortic node dissection is performed as outlined previously.

The LAVH BSO and pelvic node dissection are described together. The procedure described here will show the left side of the pelvis. Surgeon and assistant positioning will be reversed for the right side. The surgeon will be on the patient's right side (opposite of the nodes being dissected). The dissecting scissors will be in the left hand in the right lateral port. The grasping instrument will be in the right hand in the suprapubic port where the lymph nodes will be removed. The assistant will be on the patient's left side with the right hand holding the camera in the umbilical port and the left hand in the left lateral port holding either the grasper or a suction. The assistant's role is to provide traction and exposure for the surgeon.

STEP 1

Identify the round ligament and divide it where it crosses the obliterated umbilical artery (also called *the umbilical ligament*) (Fig. 4-1). Open the lateral pelvic space by incising the peritoneum lateral to the ovarian vessels up to the bifurcation of the common iliac. Maintain medial and ventral traction on the ovarian vessels so the tissue planes will be easily exposed (Fig. 4-2).

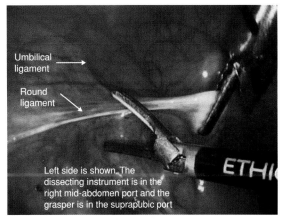

Figure 4-1. Divide the round ligament where it crosses the umbilical ligament.

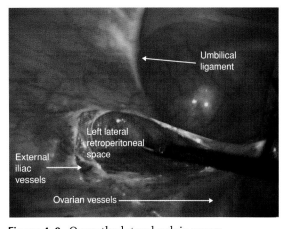

Figure 4-2. Open the lateral pelvic space.

STEP 2

Identify the ureter and separate it from the ovarian vessels. Follow it into the deep pelvis and separate it from the internal iliac vessels (Fig. 4-3).

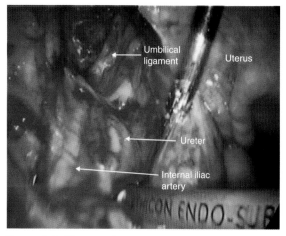

Figure 4-3. Expose the ureter.

STEP 3

Expose the contents of the left pelvic space by opening the space between the umbilical ligament and the iliac vessels. This will open the obturator space as well (Fig. 4-4).

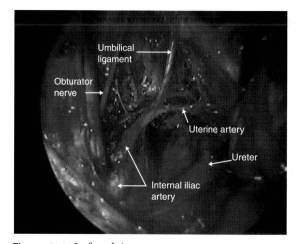

Figure 4-4. Left pelvic space open.

STEP 4

Dissect the external iliac nodes. Grasp the node chain medial to the artery with the grasper in the suprapubic port. Give medial traction while incising the fascia attached to the iliac artery from the bifurcation of the common iliac down to the distal portion of the external iliac vessels. Transect at both ends (Fig. 4-5).

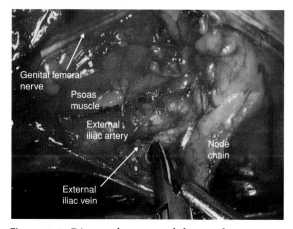

Figure 4-5. Dissect the external iliac nodes.

STEP 5

Reach directly under the external iliac vein with the suprapubic port grasper and grasp the obturator node bundle. Maintain medial traction and use the dissector to find the nerve (Fig. 4-6). The assistant uses the grasper in the left lateral port to place lateral traction on the external iliac vein. The camera should be rotated to approximately 90 degrees to better expose the space. The lymph node bundle is ventral to the nerve. The nerve is dissected away from the nodes, and the nodes are transected distally. The node bundle is dissected cephalad toward the iliac bifurcation. Here, the nerve must again be pushed lateral to avoid accidental injury (Fig. 4-7).

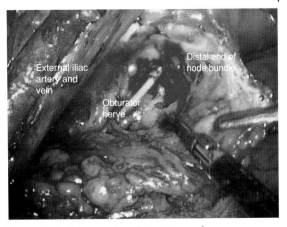

Figure 4-6. Dissect the obturator nodes.

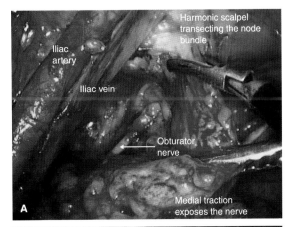

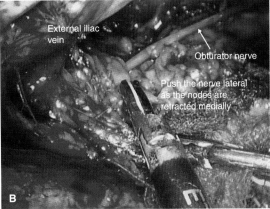

Figure 4-7. A. Cut the distal end of the obturator nodes. **B.** The obturator nerve is dissected cephalad.

The ovarian vessels are divided, and the peritoneum is incised down to the uterosacral ligaments (Fig. 4-8).

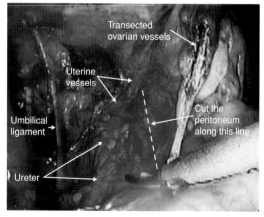

Figure 4–8. Transect the ovarian vessels and incise the peritoneum.

The bladder peritoneum is incised, and the plane between the bladder and the lower cervix and vagina is opened. Ventral traction is placed on the bladder with the suprapubic port grasper and cephalad traction on the uterus (Fig. 4-9).

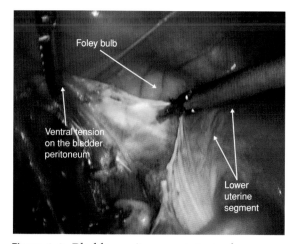

Figure 4–9. Bladder peritoneum is incised.

The hysterectomy can be completed from the vaginal side at any time. It is acceptable to perform a complete laparoscopic hysterectomy if the operator is skilled to do so. If the vagina is of adequate size, it is usually easier to finish the hysterectomy from the vagina. When the vagina is small or the patient's legs will not allow the lithotomy position, then the total laparoscopic hysterectomy is indicated.

STEP 9

When the total hysterectomy is performed, the uterine arteries are isolated and divided (Fig. 4-10). The cardinal and uterosacral ligaments are divided. Prior to entering the vagina, a mechanism to avoid release of CO_2 from the abdomen is necessary.

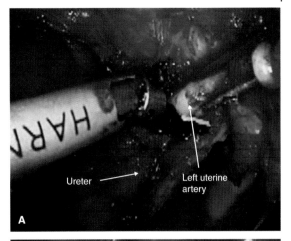

Ureter

Left uterine artery

A

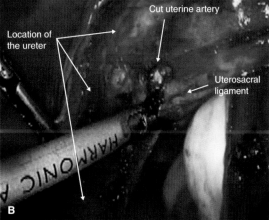

Cut uterine artery

Location of the ureter

Uterosacral ligament

B

Figure 4-10. A. Divide the left uterine artery. **B.** Divide the uterosacral ligament.

Commercially available instruments or a simple vaginal pack may be used. The uterus is separated from the vagina and removed through the vagina (Fig. 4-11). The vagina can be closed with the laparoscopic needle driver passing sutures through the suprapubic port or with commercially available instruments to pass sutures.

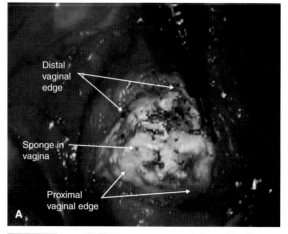

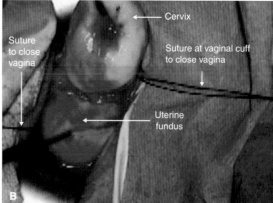

Figure 4–11. A. Cut into the vagina. **B.** Remove the uterus through the vagina.

STEP 10

When the hysterectomy is finished vaginally, the legs are brought up into the lithotomy position; adjustable stirrups will make this easy. The cervicovaginal junction is incised, and both the prevesical and prerectal spaces are entered to isolate the uterosacral and cardinal ligaments. These are clamped, cut, and tied (Fig. 4-12). The uterine arteries are isolated and clamped, cut, and tied. The uterus can now be removed. The vaginal edges are sutured for hemostasis and then closed in the midline. This reunites the cardinal and uterosacral ligaments in the midline providing more support to the vaginal apex to prevent future prolapse. The 10-mm port sites are closed to prevent hernia formation. The skin is closed with a liquid adhesive or with suture. Patients experience less pain and better scar prevention when the skin adhesive is used.

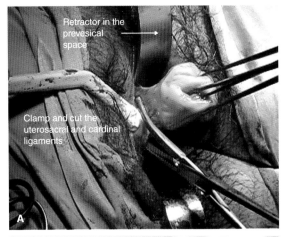

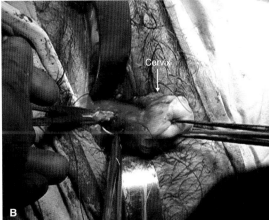

Figure 4-12. A. Clamp and cut the uterosacral and cardinal ligaments. **B.** Clamp on the uterine artery.

References

1. Childers J, Surwit E. A combined laparoscopic vaginal approach in the management of stage I endometrial cancer. *Gynecol Oncol.* 1991;45:46–51.
2. Kohler C, Tozzi R, Kelmm P, et al. Laparoscopic para-aortic left-sided transperitoneal infrarenal lymphadenectomy in patients with gynecologic malignancies: technique and results. *Gynecol Oncol.* 2003;91:139–148.
3. Spirtos NM, Eisenkop SM, Schlaerth JB, et al. Laparoscopic radical hysterectomy (type III) with aortic and pelvic lymphadenectomy in patients with stage I cervical cancer surgical morbidity and intermediate follow-up. *Am J Obstet Gynecol.* 2002;187:340–348.
4. Hertel H, Kohler C, Michels W, et al. Laparoscopic-assisted radical vaginal hysterectomy (LARVH): prospective evaluation of 200 patients with cervical cancer. *Gynecol Oncol.* 2003;90:505–511.
5. Spirtos N, Schlaerth J, Gross GM, et al. Cost and quality of life analyses of surgery for early endometrial cancer: laparotomy versus laparoscopy. *Am J Obstet Gynecol.* 1996;174:1795–1799.
6. Melendez TD, Childers JM, Nour M, et al. Laparoscopic staging of endometrial cancer: the learning experience. *J Soc Laparoendosc Surg.* 1997;1:45–49.
7. Gemignani M, Curtin J, Barakat R, et al. Laparoscopic-assisted vaginal hysterectomy (LAVH) versus total abdominal hysterectomy (TAH) for endometrial adenocarcinoma: a comparison of clinical outcomes and hospital charges [abstract]. *Gynecol Oncol.* 1998;68:129.

8. Childers J, Brzechffa P, Hatch K, et al. Laparoscopically assisted surgical staging (LASS) of endometrial cancer. *Gynecol Oncol.* 1992;51:33–38.

9. Childers J, Hatch K, Surwit E. The role of laparoscopic lymphadenectomy in the management of cervical carcinoma. *Gynecol Oncol.* 1992;47:38–43.

10. Gemignani ML, Curtin JP, Zelmanovich J, et al. Laparoscopic-assisted vaginal hysterectomy for endometrial cancer: clinical outcomes and hospital charges. *Gynecol Oncol.* 1999;73:5–11.

11. Scribner DR Jr, Mannel RS, Walker JL, et al. Cost analysis of laparoscopy versus laparotomy for early endometrial cancer. *Gynecol Oncol.* 1999;75:460–463.

12. Holub Z, Jabor A, Bartos P, et al. Laparoscopic surgery for endometrial cancer: long-term results of a multicentric study. *Eur J Gynaecol Oncol.* 2002;23:305–310.

13. Khosia I, Lowe C. Indices of obesity derived from body weight and height. *Br J Prev Med Soc.* 1967;21:122–123.

14. Holub Z, Bartos P, Jabor A, et al. Laproscopic surgery in obese women with endometrial cancer. *J Am Assoc Gynecol Laparosc.* 2000;7:83–88.

15. Eltabbakh GH, Shamonki MI, Moody JM, et al. Hysterectomy for obese women with endometrial cancer: laparoscopy or laparotomy? *Gynecol Oncol.* 2000;78:329–335.

16. Eltabbakh GH. Analysis of survival after laparoscopy in women with endometrial carcinoma. *Cancer.* 2002;95:1894–1901.

17. Malur S, Possover M, Michels W, et al. *Gynecol Oncol.* 2001;80:239–244.

18. Hatch KD. Clinical outcomes and long term survival after laparoscopic staging and hysterectomy for endometrial cancer [abstract]. 2004 SGO Abstract, 2004.

19. Holub Z, Jabor A, Kliment L. Comparison of two procedures for sentinel lymph node detection in patients with endometrial cancer: a pilot study. *Eur J Gynaecol Oncol.* 2002;23:53–57.

20. Gargiulo T, Giusti M, Bottero A, et al. Sentinel lymphnode (SLN) laparoscopic assessment in early stage endometrial cancer. *Minerva Gynecol.* 2008;55:259–262.

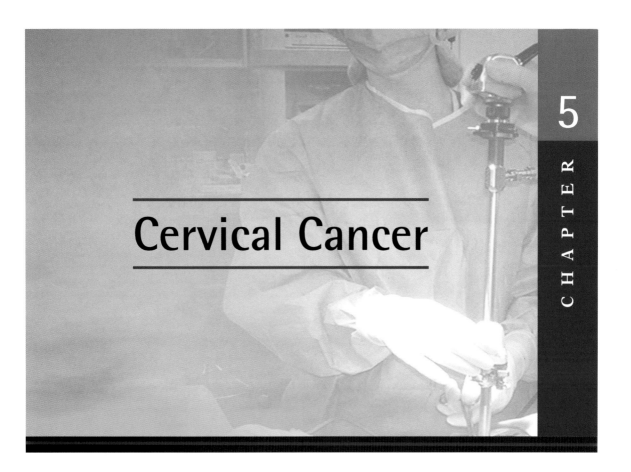

Cervical Cancer

The use of laparoscopy in the treatment of cervical cancer has been limited by the fact that there did not appear to be an advantage to laparoscopic lymphadenectomy because the standard operation for the primary cervical tumor has been radical abdominal hysterectomy.

Dargent (1) first suggested that laparoscopic pelvic lymphadenectomy could be followed by a Schauta radical vaginal hysterectomy and has published the only long-term results of such a procedure. The 3-year survival rate of 51 patients with negative pelvic lymph nodes was 95.5%. Querleu (2) reported eight patients and demonstrated an average blood loss of <300 mL, an average hospital stay of 4.2 days, and decreased pain from the elimination of an abdominal or perineal incision. Hatch et al. (3) reported 37 patients treated by laparoscopic pelvic and para-aortic lymphadenectomy followed by radical vaginal hysterectomy. The mean operative time was 225 minutes, the mean blood loss was 525 mL, and the average hospital stay was 3 days. Blood transfusion was required in 11% of the patients, compared with the range of 35% to 95% reported in the literature for radical abdominal hysterectomy. Complications occurred early in the series and included two cystotomies repaired at surgery without an increase in hospital stay or further complications. In two patients (5.4%), ureterovaginal fistulas developed that were treated by ureteral stents, which were removed 6 weeks later without further operative intervention.

Schneider et al. (4) reported on 33 patients in whom bipolar techniques were used for lymphadenectomy and to transect the cardinal ligaments and uterine vessels. Hysterectomy was completed by the Schauta-Stoeckel technique. There were five (15%) intraoperative injuries managed successfully without subsequent sequelae. Four patients required transfusion. Roy et al. (5) reported 52 patients in whom laparoscopic pelvic lymphadenectomy was followed by a radical vaginal hysterectomy in 25 cases or a radical abdominal hysterectomy in 27 cases. The two groups were comparable in blood loss (400 mL vs. 450 mL), operating time (270 minutes vs. 280 minutes), blood transfusion (five patients vs. four patients), and postoperative stay (7 days for both groups). There was an increase in febrile morbidity, wound infection, and ileus in the patients having abdominal radical hysterectomy. With a mean follow-up of 27 months, only one recurrence has been noted.

Recent studies have shown that the complication rates go down as the operator experience increases (6,7). Long-term survival is reported by Hertel et al. (8) in 200 patients with a mean follow-up of 40 months; the projected 5-year survival was 83%. For the 100 patients who were stage 1, lymphvascular space node negative the survival was 98%.

Technique

Laparoscopic Assisted Radical Vaginal Hysterectomy

Preoperative Preparation

The patient preparation begins with a clear liquid diet the day before the surgical procedure. The patient is given a laxative to evacuate the bowel. It is important for the bowel to be collapsed during lymphadenectomy so that the proper exposure can be obtained.

Operative Approach

The patient is positioned in the dorsal lithotomy position with the legs in stirrups, which support the leg and decrease the tension on the femoral and peroneal nerves. The arms are tucked at each side, an orogastric tube is in place, and a Foley catheter is in the urethra.

A 10- to 12-mm trocar is inserted into the umbilicus. Additional trocars are placed in the right and left lower quadrants just lateral to the inferior epigastric vessels. A 10- to 12-mm trocar is placed in the suprapubic site so that the lymph nodes can be removed through the port. The patient is placed in the Trendelenburg position to help pack the bowel into the upper abdomen.

The principles of laparoscopic surgery are similar to those of laparotomy. There must be adequate exposure, identification of anatomy, and removal of the appropriate structures. Sponges or mini laparotomy packs can be placed around loops of bowel to aid in exposure and to block small amounts of blood. This decreases the necessity for a suction apparatus in the abdomen and allows the port to be used as graspers or cautery.

The para-aortic node dissection will be performed first when the cancer is ≥2 cm. The right aortic nodes are sampled first. The left side is usually performed as well; however, this will depend upon the surgeon's philosophy on the surgical management of cervical cancer. If the surgeon would normally remove the left para-aortic nodes in an open case, then it should be done laparoscopically as well.

FIGURE 1

The peritoneum is incised between the sigmoid mesentery and the small bowel mesentery up to the duodenum. The node chain is isolated and dissection is carried out. Monopolar surgery, bipolar surgery, harmonic scalpel, and argon beam coagulator have all been successfully used. The landmarks for dissection are the reflection of the duodenum, the inferior mesentery artery superiorly, and the psoas muscles laterally (Fig. 5-1).

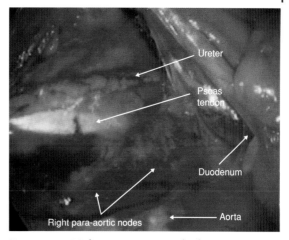

Figure 5-1. Right para-aortic node dissection.

STEP 1

The ureter must be identified and placed on traction by the assistant to keep it out of the operative field. Common iliac nodes can be exposed through the retroperitoneal incision made from the para-aortic node dissection site (Fig. 5-2). It is possible to resect the upper portion of the common iliac nodes from this approach, and the remainders of the common iliac nodes are dissected from the pelvic node incision sites.

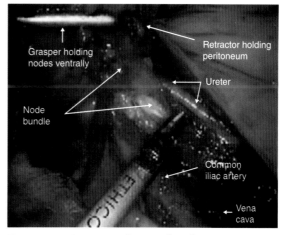

Figure 5-2. Common iliac nodes from para-aortic exposure.

STEP 2

The pelvic node dissection is begun by dividing the round ligaments and finding the lateral pelvic space (Fig. 5-3). The obliterated umbilical artery is retracted medialward opening up the entire lateral pelvic space.

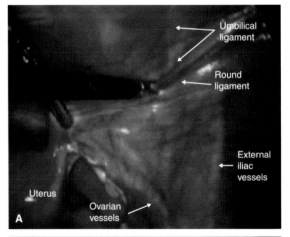

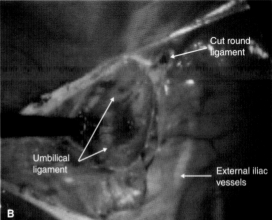

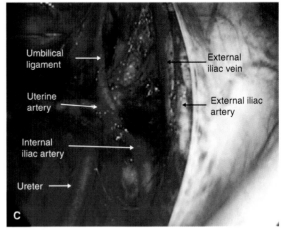

Figure 5-3. A. Open right pelvic space by opening right round ligament. **B.** Enter the lateral pelvic space lateral to the umbilical ligament. **C.** Right pelvic anatomy.

STEP 3

An entire lymphadenectomy is performed, including the nodes between the iliac vessels and psoas muscle. The entire obturator space is dissected.

STEP 4

The lymph nodes medial to the external iliac artery are placed on traction with the left hand grasper in the suprapubic port. The dissecting instrument is in the right hand in the lateral port for a dissection on the patient's right side. The fascial attachments of the nodes to the artery are incised medial to the artery (Fig. 5-4).

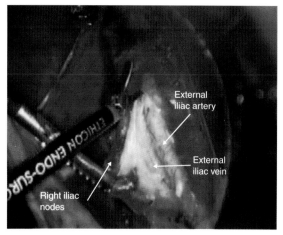

Figure 5-4. Right external iliac node dissection.

STEP 5

The dissection proceeds caudad to the femoral canal. The medial chain of the external iliac nodes is divided there, and the dissection proceeds cephalad to the common iliac vessels. The nodes are transected and removed (Fig. 5-5).

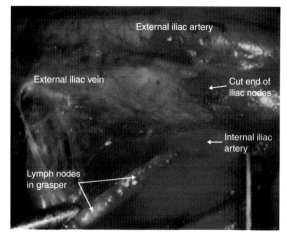

Figure 5-5. External iliac nodes dissected over the vein.

STEP 6

The lateral external nodes are dissected starting lateral to the common iliac artery. The genital femoral nerve is the lateral boundary. The
space between the iliac vessels and the psoas
muscle is developed. The upper lateral obturator space is visible from this position. Any
lymph nodes left in this space can be removed
(Fig. 5-6).

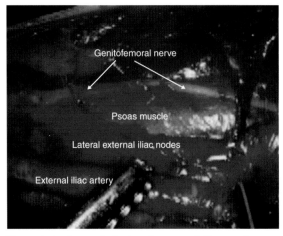

Figure 5-6. Lateral chain of external iliac nodes.

STEP 7

The common iliac nodes are removed by further opening the space between the common
iliac and the psoas cephalad. These nodes are
lateral to the common iliac. The para-aortic
node dissection site will be the upper boundary
of this dissection (Fig. 5-7).

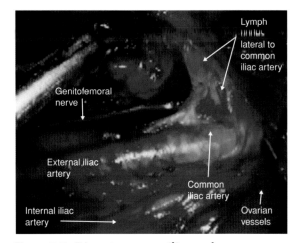

Figure 5-7. Dissect common iliac nodes.

STEP 8

The obturator nodes are removed by grasping the node bundle directly under the iliac vein. The nerve is identified and retracted laterally (Fig. 5-8).

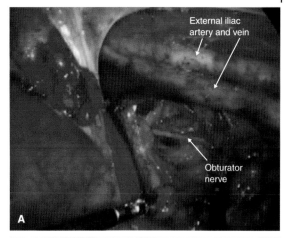

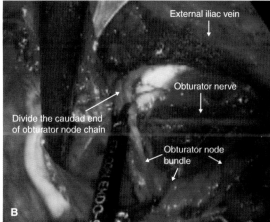

Figure 5-8. Exposing the right obturator nerve.

STEP 9

The node bundle is dissected caudad and divided. The bundle is placed on traction medial and ventral as it is dissected cephalad. The node bundle is transected at the level of the bifurcation of the common iliac artery. The obturator nerve must be retracted laterally during this dissection to avoid accidental injury (Fig. 5-9).

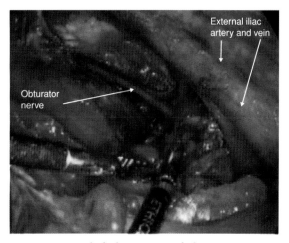

Figure 5-9. Cephalad exposure of obturator nerve.

STEP 10

Following the complete pelvic lymphadenectomy, the paravesical and pararectal spaces are open. The uterine artery is identified and isolated at its origin (Fig. 5-10). It is then divided and brought up and over the ureter. The uterine vein is transected and mobilized medially. The lateral attachments of the cardinal ligament are dissected away from the internal iliac vessels (Fig. 5-11).

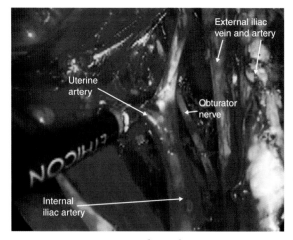

Figure 5-10. Transecting the right uterine artery.

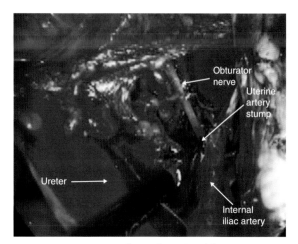

Figure 5-11. Transect lateral cardinal ligament.

STEP 11

It is important to identify and preserve the hypogastric nerve in order to preserve normal bladder and bowel function. If the para-aortic nodes have been dissected the superior hypogastric plexus is exposed at the bifurcation of the aorta (Fig. 5-12).

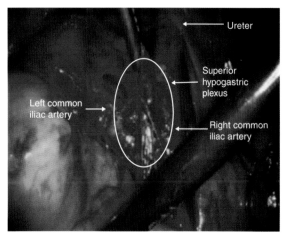

Figure 5-12. Superior hypogastric plexus at the bifurcation of the aorta.

FIGURE 13

The hypogastric nerve is identified at the pelvic brim by opening the peritoneum medial to the ureter (Fig. 5-13).

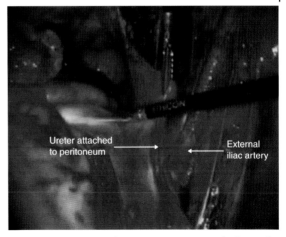

Figure 5-13. Open the peritoneum medial to the ureter.

FIGURE 14

Placing traction on the nerve will show its course from the pelvic brim into the pelvis (Fig. 5-14).

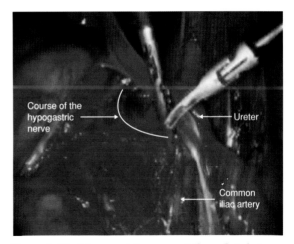

Figure 5-14. Hypogastric nerve at the pelvic brim.

FIGURE 15

The ureter is retracted medially, and the hypogastric nerve in the mid-pelvis is identified (Fig. 5-15).

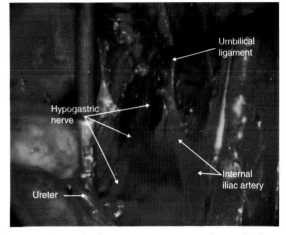

Figure 5-15. The hypogastric nerve in the midpelvis.

FIGURE 16

The nerve enters the cardinal ligament dorsal and lateral to the ureter and deep to the cut uterine artery (Fig. 5-16).

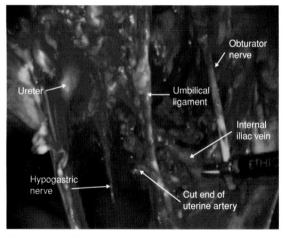

Figure 5-16. Hypogastric nerve lateral and dorsal to the ureter.

FIGURE 17

Its location to the uterine artery and vein are demonstrated (Fig. 5-17).

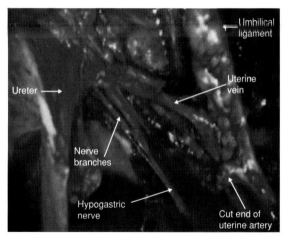

Figure 5-17. Location of the nerve in cardinal ligament.

FIGURE 18

The ureter is dissected off the uterosacral ligament (Fig. 5-18).

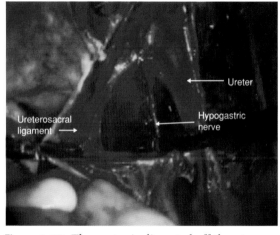

Figure 5-18. The ureter is dissected off the uterosacral ligament.

STEP 12

The peritoneum over the uterosacral ligament is divided at the level of the rectum. The ligament is sharply dissected and with the aid of the harmonic scalpel or electrosurgical cautery to drop the rectum away from the uterosacral ligaments (Fig. 5-19).

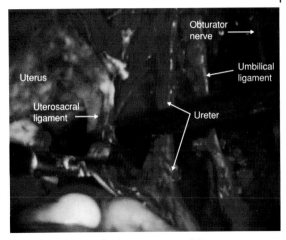

Figure 5-19. Divide the uterosacral ligament.

STEP 13

The bladder flap has been advanced and the vesicouterine ligament is sharply divided using harmonic scalpel (Fig. 5-20).

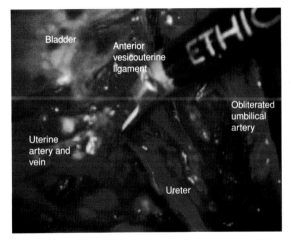

Figure 5-20. Divide the anterior vesicouterine ligament.

STEP 14

The surgical procedure then moves to the vaginal side. The legs are brought up into the lithotomy position and the cervix is exposed. Diluted epinephrine solution (1–100,000) is injected circumferentially under the vaginal mucosa, approximately 3 cm from cervical vaginal junction and the incision is made (Fig. 5-21).

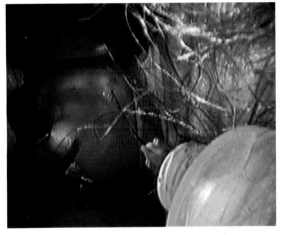

Figure 5-21. Inject vasoconstrictor agent into vagina.

STEP 15

The prevesical space is developed and a curved retractor is placed. The vaginal mucosa in the posterior cul-de-sac incised, and the rectum is dropped away (Fig. 5-22).

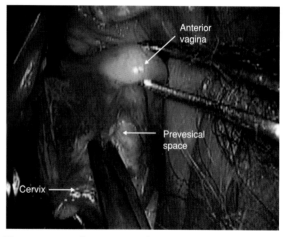

Figure 5-22. The prevesical space is developed.

STEP 16

The bladder pillar is developed by grasping the vaginal mucosa at approximately 3 o'clock position; the Metzenbaum scissors are used to dissect submucosally until the paravesical space is entered. This is enlarged so that a Brisky retractor can be placed. This then isolates the bladder pillar from the cardinal ligaments (Fig. 5-23).

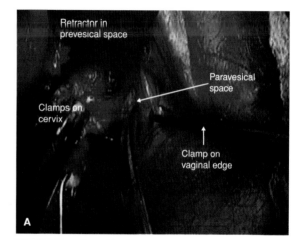

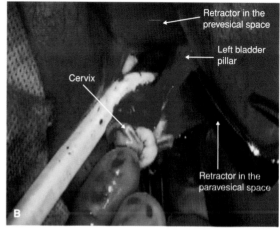

Figure 5-23. A. Entering the left paravesical space. **B.** Retractors isolate the bladder pillars.

STEP 17

The cardinal ligament attachments to the vagina are clamped at the sidewall, divided, and ligated. This allows for greater mobility of the uterus and easier dissection of the ureter in the bladder pillar (Fig. 5-24).

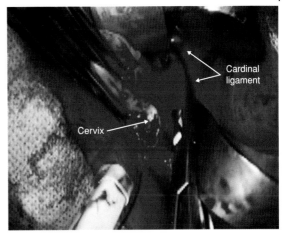

Figure 5-24. Clamp on the left cardinal ligament.

STEP 18

The bladder pillar is then divided into a medial and later portion. The ureter is found at the midportion of the bladder pillar (Fig. 5-25). The ureter undergoes a sharp bend at this point and as it is dissected out the uterine, vessels become visible (Fig. 5-26). The vessels are then brought under the ureter, and the ureter is freed from the rest of the attachments and pushed cephalad. Usually, there are further peritoneal attachments that need to be divided, and the specimen can be removed.

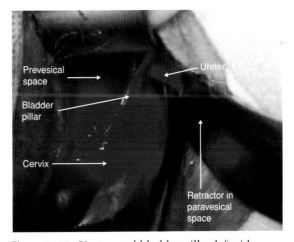

Figure 5-25. Ureter and bladder pillar left side.

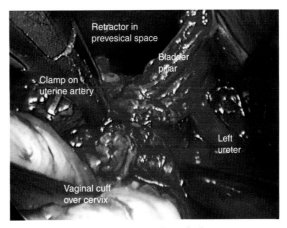

Figure 5-26. Uterine artery identified.

STEP 19

After hemostasis is assured, the peritoneum from the bladder is sewn to the anterior edge of the vaginal mucosa (Fig. 5-27). The peritoneum from the cul-de-sac over the rectum is sewn to the posterior vaginal mucosa. This allows from greater length of the vagina to be established by inward migration of the squamous epithelium.

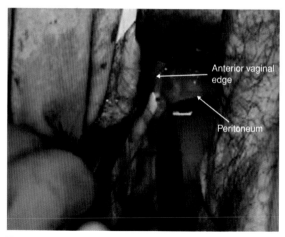

Figure 5-27. Anterior peritoneum sewn to anterior vagina edge.

STEP 20

The CO_2 is reinsufflated and the pelvis is inspected for hemostasis and for any unsuspected injuries to the bladder or ureter (Fig. 5-28). The pelvis is irrigated and the 10- to 12-mm trocar sites are closed with absorbable suture. The CO_2 is allowed to escape and the skin is closed with 4-0 absorbable suture or skin adhesive. Marcaine is injected in the skin incision sited to decrease postoperative pain.

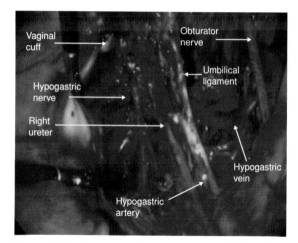

Figure 5-28. Postoperative appearance of the pelvis.

Postoperative Management

Patients are given a clear liquid diet the night of the surgery and a regular diet the morning after surgery. They are generally able to be discharged on the second or third postoperative day. Complications of laparoscopy for malignant disease are higher than for benign disease. Postoperative complications of wound infection, ileus, and fever occur, but at lower rates than after laparotomy. Adynamic ileus is unusual after laparoscopic surgery, but any abdominal distention, worsening of pain, or vomiting must be taken seriously. Unsuspected bowel injuries manifest themselves by abdominal distention, pain, and free air. The carbon dioxide used for insufflation should be absorbed within hours, so any free air in the abdomen is highly suspicious of perforation. Data on complication rates from laparoscopic lymphadenectomy are inadequate due to small sample sizes, lack of adjustment for a learning curve, and confounding by combinations of and differences in procedures. We have not observed postoperative lymphocyst formation in over 140 cases.

Laparoscopic lymphadenectomy followed by radical vaginal hysterectomy is an excellent option for patients with stage IA or IB cancer of the cervix. Compared with radical abdominal hysterectomy and lymphadenectomy, it has less blood loss, fewer hospital days, and more rapid return to full activity with comparable survival.

Laparoscopic Radical Hysterectomy

Although most reports in the literature have detailed some form of laparoscopically assisted radical vaginal hysterectomy, there also are reports of laparoscopic radical hysterectomy. Nezhat et al. (9) and Canis et al. (10) have reported laparoscopic radical hysterectomy in separate case reports. Spirtos et al. (11) reported laparoscopic radical hysterectomy with aortic and pelvic lymphadenectomy in 78 patients. The average operative time was 205 minutes, length of hospitalization was 3.2 days, and blood loss was 225 mL; one transfusion was necessary. There were acceptable intraoperative and postoperative complications with a minimum of 3-year follow-up the diseasefree survival is 95%.

The issue of blood loss and transfusion has become very important to patients and surgeons since the identification of the human immunodeficiency virus. Every report on laparoscopic lymphadenectomy and radical hysterectomy has noted a significant decrease in blood loss and transfusion rates. Other societal advantages are the decreased hospital stay and rapid return to normal function, even with radical surgery.

Laparoscopic staging of cervical cancer prior to treatment planning has been proposed (9,12,13). Vidaurreta et al. (12) staged 91 stage IIb, IIIab and IVb patients computed tomography (CT) was performed in 49 patients: 38 read as normal and 11 as positive. Histologic evaluation revealed metastases in 18 of the 38 negative scan patients and no metastases were found in five of the 11 with positive scans. Hertel et al. (13) compared laparoscopic surgical staging to findings of magnetic resonance imaging (MRI) and CT scans in 101 patients; 91 of whom had CT scans; 67 had MRI; and 49 had both. False-positive or false-negative results were found in 22% of patients. In 10 patients who were false positive for para-aortic node metastasis, extended field radiotherapy had been planned and was canceled, which significantly reduced the patient's morbidity.

Technique

Laparoscopic Radical Hysterectomy

The laparoscopic radical hysterectomy is performed by performing steps 1 to 14 for the laparoscopic assisted radical vaginal hysterectomy. After step 14, the procedure does not go to the vaginal side; instead, the following steps are performed.

STEP 1

The uterine artery is brought over the ureter. The vesicouterine ligaments are divided to their insertion into the vagina. The ureter is dissected completely out of the cardinal ligament to the trigone (Fig. 5-29).

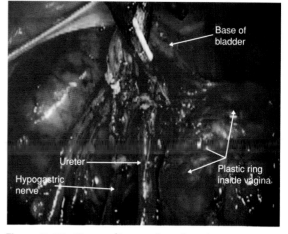

Figure 5-29. Ureter dissected to the trigone.

STEP 2

The upper vagina is entered by dissection with the Harmonic scalpel (Fig. 5-30). A manipulator placed in the vagina and uterus that has a cup fitting around the cervix provides the traction needed to assist vaginal entry.

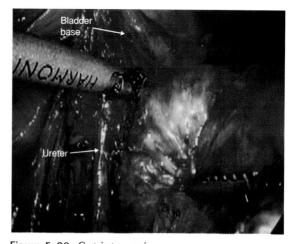

Figure 5-30. Cut into vagina.

STEP 3

The specimen is pulled out of the vagina. The vagina is closed using the same techniques as in the laparoscopic assisted radical vaginal hysterectomy.

Table 5-1 **Sentinel Node for Cervical Cancer**

Reference	No.	Sentinel Nodes (%)	Sensitivity	Negative	Detection
Dargent (14)	35	85	100		Blue dye
Lantzsch (15)	14	93	100	100	Tech
Malur (16)	50	78	83	97	Tech plus blue dye
Levenback (17)	30	100	87.5	97	Tech plus blue dye
Buist (18)	25	100	89	90	Tech plus blue dye
Lambaudie (19)	12	100	66	90	Tech plus blue dye

Tech, Technetium 99m.

Sentinel Nodes

The initial studies of detection of sentinel nodes showed sensitivity, negative predictive value, and accuracy of 100%. Dargent et al. (14), Lantzsch et al. (15), and Malur et al. (16) reported 100% sensitivity and negative predictive value, but only when both blue dye and Technetium 99m were used. Subsequent studies have used both detection methods with varying success (Table 5-1).

Radical Vaginal Trachelectomy

In 1994, Dargent et al. (20) first presented a series of 28 patients who underwent laparoscopic pelvic lymphadenectomy followed by radical vaginal trachelectomy. After a median follow-up of 36 months, there was only one recurrence in the para-aortic nodes of a 27-year-old woman with stage IB adenocarcinoma: The pelvic lymph nodes had been negative and the margins were free. Among the eight patients who desired pregnancy, three had cesarean section at 36 weeks' gestation, and three had spontaneous abortions. The second report on radical vaginal trachelectomy was published in 1998 by Roy and Plante (21). Thirty patients underwent laparoscopic pelvic lymphadenectomy and radical vaginal trachelectomy; only six women had attempted pregnancy at the time of reporting, and four had healthy infants delivered by cesarean section.

A number of authors have now reported their experience with radical trachelectomy (Table 5-2). The indications commonly used are: (a) desire for future childbearing, (b) lesion ≤2 cm in size, (c) no involvement of upper endocervix by colposcopy, MRI or intraoperative frozen section, (d) no metastasis to regional lymph nodes, (e) for stage IAI lesions, lymphvascular space invasion should be present.

There have been no recurrences in the uterus. The risk factors for recurrence are lesion size >2 cm, depth of invasion >1 cm, and lymphvascular space invasion (25).

Table 5-2 **Outcomes Following Radical Vaginal Trachelectomy**

	Plante (22)	Covens (22)	Dargent (24,25) Bernardini (23)	Shepherd (26)	Burnett (27)	Schlaerth (28)	Total
Cases	68	80/93[a]	82	26	19	10	298
Follow-up	34	30	76	23	31	47	40
Months	(1–144)	(1–103)	(NS)	(1–64)	(22–44)	(28–84)	
Recurrences	1 (1.5%)	7 (7.3%)	3 (3.6%)	0	0	0	11 (3.6%)
Pregnancies Women	33/23	22/18	47/29	14/8	3/3	4/4	123/85
Deliveries	24	18	27	9	2	2	82 (67%)

[a]Oncology outcome based on 93 cases; pregnancy outcome based on 80 cases.

Overall, 67% of 85 women having 123 pregnancies delivered viable pregnancies. The first-trimester abortion rate was 17%, which is similar to the general population. The second-trimester rate was 12%, which is much higher than expected. Of the viable pregnancies, 10% to 15% were born between 24 and 28 weeks' gestation. Therefore, pregnancies should be managed by maternal fetal medicine specialists.

Technique

Pelvic Lymph Node Dissection and Radical Trachelectomy for Early Cervical Cancer

Women with early cervical cancer who want to preserve their childbearing ability may benefit from this operation. The pelvic lymph nodes will be dissected as if doing a radical hysterectomy. The cardinal ligament will be removed while preserving the uterine vessels, uterine fundus and the adnexa. The patient preparation and positioning are the same as for any radical gynecologic procedure.

The right pelvic dissection is shown.

STEP 1

The round ligament is preserved. The peritoneum lateral to the ovarian vessels is incised from the round ligament to the pelvic brim. The ovarian vessels are preserved (Fig. 5-31).

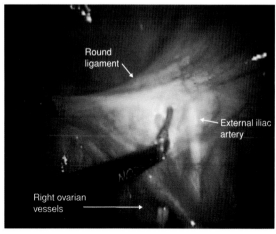

Figure 5-31. Open lateral to the ovarian vessels.

STEP 2

Perform the lymph node dissection as described before removing all the nodes from the obturator space and up to the common iliac.

STEP 3

Develop the pararectal space. Place the umbilical ligament on traction and make a window just cephalad to the uterine artery at its origin from the internal iliac artery (Fig. 5-32). Open this space widely to get good visualization of the cardinal ligament contents.

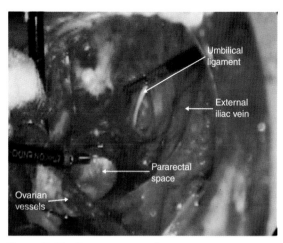

Figure 5-32. Open pararectal space.

STEP 4

Develop the paravesical space. The ureter will stay on the peritoneum medially and the internal iliac artery will be lateral. The cardinal ligament contents are now fully exposed (Fig. 5-33).

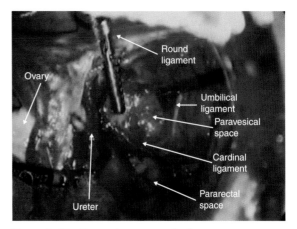

Figure 5-33. Open the paravesical space.

STEP 5

The uterine vessels are mobilized and left intact. The lateral cardinal ligament will be removed with sharp and blunt dissection. The harmonic scalpel will be the safest instrument to use here because of its low temperature and reliable vessel sealing (Fig. 5-34).

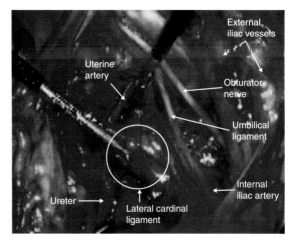

Figure 5-34. Remove lateral cardinal ligament nodes.

STEP 6

Removing the lateral cardinal ligament contents will expose the internal iliac vessels (Fig. 5-35).

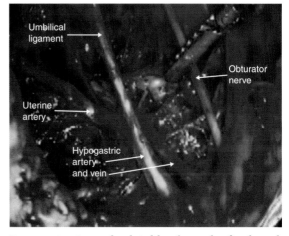

Figure 5-35. Lateral pelvic blood vessels after lymph node dissection.

STEP 7

The medial cardinal ligament will be removed from the vaginal side. To make it easier and safer, further mobilize the uterine artery and the ureter, begin the ureteral tunnel and elevate the uterine vessels away from it (Fig. 5-36).

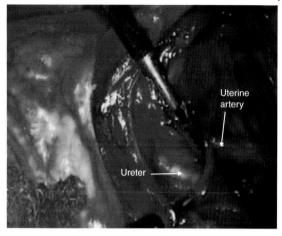

Figure 5-36. Ureter tunnel is dissected.

STEP 8

The operation goes to the vaginal side. The vaginal incision will be made 2 cm from the cervical vaginal junction. The prevesical space will be developed but the peritoneum will not be entered (Figs. 5-21 and 5-22).

STEP 9

The bladder pillars are isolated similar to the radical vaginal hysterectomy (Fig. 5-23). This separates the bladder pillar from the cardinal ligament.

STEP 10

The posterior vagina is opened into the peritoneal cavity. With the Brisky retractors in place, the uterosacral and cardinal ligaments can be clamped 2 to 3 cm from the cervix. This allows the bladder pillars to descend and makes it easier to dissect the ureters.

STEP 11

The left ureter is exposed by leaving the Brisky retractor in its 2 o'clock position, placing the left index finger into the midline of the pre-vesical space, and palpating the bladder pillar by pushing against the Brisky retractor (Fig. 5-37). The ureter is a firm cordlike structure that rolls over the finger and makes an almost audible "click."

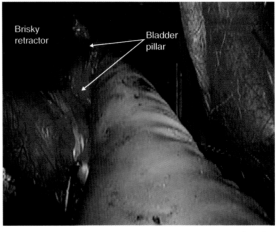

Figure 5-37. Finger palpating ureter in the bladder pillar.

STEP 12

The bladder pillar is then divided into a medial and lateral portion (Fig. 5-38). The lateral portion is dissected first, as this is avascular. This is sharply divided and the ureter is seen. It is dissected cephalad from the lateral side to expose the length of the tunnel (Fig. 5-39).

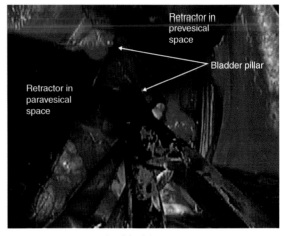

Figure 5-38. Split the bladder pillar.

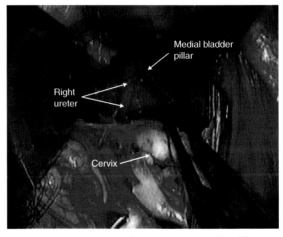

Figure 5-39. Exposing the ureter in the bladder pillar.

STEP 13

The ureter is mobilized laterally to expose the uterine artery, which will be medial and cephalad. The ureter is retracted 1 cm lateral, and the descending portion of the uterine artery is clamped and divided (Fig. 5-40).

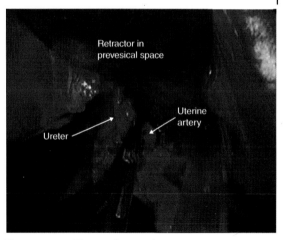

Figure 5-40. Clamp the uterine artery.

STEP 14

The right side is dissected.

STEP 15

A uterine dilator is placed into the cervix and the location of the internal os is identified. The location of the ligated uterine arteries should also be at this level.

STEP 16

The cervix is transected (Fig. 5-41). A frozen section of the apex is obtained. A small biopsy from the remaining upper edge of the cervix is sent for frozen. If either specimen has invasive cancer, then additional tissue will have to be removed or the patient should have a hysterectomy.

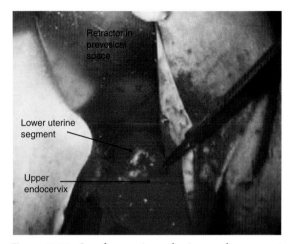

Figure 5-41. Cut the cervix at the internal os.

STEP 17

A cerclage is placed around the lower uterine segment to help prevent premature delivery (Fig. 5-42).

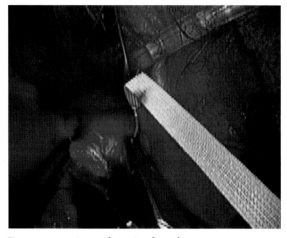

Figure 5-42. A cerclage is placed.

STEP 18

The vagina is attached to the uterine stump with running suture (Figs. 5-43 and 5-44).

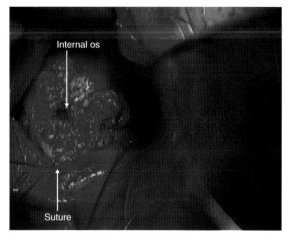

Figure 5-43. Sew the vagina to the uterus.

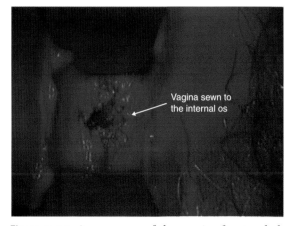

Figure 5-44. Appearance of the cervix after trachelectomy.

STEP 19

A Foley catheter is placed over night. Most patients are discharged on day 1 or 2.

STEP 20

The patients are seen every 2 weeks to place a probe into the canal to decrease stricture. The first Pap smear is performed at 4 months.

References

1. Dargent D. A new future for Schauta's operation through a presurgical retroperitoneal pelviscopy. *Eur J Gynaecol Oncol*. 1987;8:292–296.
2. Scribner DR Jr, Mannel RS, Walker JL, et al. Cost analysis of laparoscopy versus laparotomy for early endometrial cancer. *Gynecol Oncol*. 1999;75:460–463.
3. Hatch KD, Hallum AV III, Nour M. New surgical approaches to treatment of cervical cancer. *J Natl Cancer Inst Monogr*. 1996;21:71–75.
4. Schneider A, Possover M, Kamprath S, et al. Laparoscopy-assisted radical vaginal hysterectomy modified according to Schauta-Stoeckel. *Obstet Gynecol*. 1996;88:1057–1060.
5. Roy M, Plante M, Renaud MC, et al. Vaginal radical hysterectomy versus abdominal radical hysterectomy in the treatment of early-stage cervical cancer. *Gynecol Oncol*. 1996;62:336–339.
6. Renaud MC, Plante M, Roy M. Combined laparoscopic and vaginal radical surgery in cervical cancer. *Gynecol Oncol*. 2000;79:59–63.
7. Querleu D, Narducci F, Poulard V, et al. Modified radical vaginal hysterectomy with or without laparoscopic nerve-sparing dissection: a comparative study. *Gynecol Oncol*. 2002;85:154–158.
8. Hertel H, Kohler C, Michels W, et al. Laparoscopic-assisted radical vaginal hysterectomy (LARVH): prospective evaluation of 200 patients with cervical cancer. *Gynecol Oncol*. 2003;90:505–511.
9. Nezhat C, Nezhat F, Burrell MO, et al. Laparoscopic radical hysterectomy with para-aortic and pelvic node dissection. *Am J Obstet Gynecol*. 1994;170–699.
10. Canis M, Mage G, Wattiez A, et al. Vaginally assisted laparoscopic radical hysterectomy. *J Gynecol Surg*. 1992;8:103–104.
11. Spirtos NM, Eisenkop SM, Schlaerth JB, et al. Laparoscopic radical hysterectomy (type III) with aortic and pelvic lymphadenectomy in patients with stage I cervical cancer surgical morbidity and intermediate follow-up. *Am J Obstet Gynoncol*. 2002;187:340–348.
12. Vidaurreta J, Bermudez A, di Paola G, et al. Laparoscopic staging in locally advanced cervical carcinoma: A new possible philosophy? *Gynecol Oncol*. 1999;75:366–371.
13. Hertel H, Kohler C, Elhawary T, et al. Laparoscopic staging compared with imaging techniques in the staging of advanced cervical cancer. *Gynecol Oncol*. 2002;87:46–51.
14. Dargent D, Martin X, Mathevet P. Laparoscopic assessment of the sentinel lymph node in early stage cervical cancer. *Gynecol Oncol*. 2000;79:411–415.
15. Lantzsch T, Wolters M, Grimm J, et al. Sentinel node procedure in Ib cervical cancer: a preliminary series. *Br J Cancer*. 2001;85:791–794.
16. Malur S, Krause N, Kohler C, et al. Sentinel lymph node detection in patients with cervical cancer. *Gynecol Oncol*. 2001;80:254–257.
17. Levenback C, Coleman RL, Burke TW, et al. Lymphatic mapping and sentinel node identification in patients with cervix cancer undergoing radical hysterectomy and pelvic lymphadenectomy. *J Clin Oncol*. 2002;20:688–693.
18. Buist MR, Pijpers RJ, van Lingen A, et al. Laparoscopic detection of sentinel lymph nodes followed by lymph node dissection in patients with early stage cervical cancer. *Gynecol Oncol*. 2003;90:290–296.

19. Lambaudie E, Collinet P, Narducci F, et al. Laparoscopic identification of sentinel lymph nodes in early stage cervical cancer: prospective study using a combination of patent blue dye injection and technetium radiocolloid injection. *Gynecol Oncol.* 2003;89:84–87.

20. Dargent D, Brun J, Roy M, et al. Pregnancies following radical trachelectomy for invasive cervical cancer [abstract]. *Gynecol Oncol.* 1994;52:105.

21. Roy M, Plante M. Pregnancies after radical vaginal trachelectomy for early stage cervical cancer. *Am J Obstet Gynecol.* 1998;179:1491–1496.

22. Plante M. Fertility preservation in the management of cervical cancer. *CME J Gynecol Oncol.* 2003;97–107.

23. Bernardini M, Barrett J, Seaward G, et al. Pregnancy outcomes in patients after radical trachelectomy. *Am J Obstet Gynecol.* 2003;189:1378–1382.

24. Dargent D. [Radical trachelectomy: an operation that preserves the fertility of young women with invasive cervical cancer]. *Bull Acad Natl Med.* 2001;185:1295–1304.

25. Dargent D, Franzosi F, Ansquer Y, et al. [Extended trachelectomy relapse: plea for patient involvement in the medical decision.] *Bull Cancer.* 2002;89:1027–1030.

26. Shepher JH, Mould T, Oram DH. Radical trachelectomy in early stage carcinoma of the cervix: outcome as judged by recurrence and fertility rates. *Br J Obstet Gyn.* 2001;108:882–885.

27. Burnett AF, Roman LD, O'Meara AT, et al. Radical vaginal trachelectomy and pelvic lymphadenectomy for preservation of fertility in early cervical carcinoma. *Gynecol Oncol.* 2003;88:419–423.

28. Schlaerth JB, Spirtos NM, Schlaerth AC. Radical trachelectomy and pelvic lymphadenectomy with uterine preservation in the treatment of cervical cancer. *Am J Obstet Gynecol.* 2003;188:29–34.

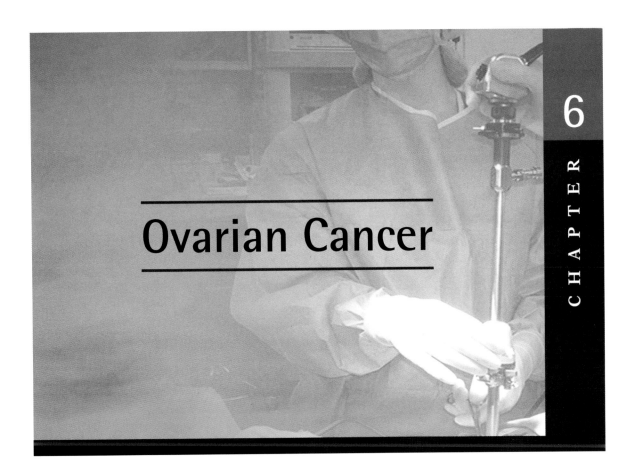

Ovarian Cancer

C H A P T E R

6

Laparoscopy has been used since the 1970's to manage adnexal masses and as a second-look procedure to avoid laparotomy in patients with persistent disease after primary chemotherapy. More recently, it has been reported to be useful for staging apparently early cancer of the ovary. The ability to perform retroperitoneal evaluation has seen it advocated again for second-look procedures.

Evaluation of the Suspicious Adnexal Mass

Laparotomy is accepted as the standard of care for management of the suspicious adnexal mass. However, it is possible to mismanage adnexal masses regardless of whether laparotomy or laparoscopy is used.

The incidence with which an unexpected malignancy is encountered when managing adnexal masses is reported to be between 0.4% and 2.9% (1–3). Childers et al. (4) and Canis et al. (5) used laparoscopy for management of suspicious adnexal masses and reported malignancy rates of 14% and 15%, respectively, and >80% of the masses were managed by laparoscopy. All of the malignancies were properly diagnosed and treated, including 13 staged by laparoscopy. It is important to perform a frozen-section analysis so that surgical staging and appropriate treatment are not delayed. Staging requires an infracolic omentectomy, peritoneal washings, multiple biopsies from the peritoneal surfaces and right hemidiaphragm, and pelvic and para-aortic lymph node biopsies.

Several investigators have reported their experiences with staging of early ovarian cancer. Querleu and LeBlanc (6) described the first adequate laparoscopic surgical staging for ovarian carcinoma. Eight patients underwent laparoscopic para-aortic lymph node sampling up to the level of the renal veins. The number of para-aortic lymph nodes per patient ranged from 6 to 17. Childers et al. (7) reported 14 patients undergoing staging for presumed early ovarian cancer. Metastatic disease was discovered in eight (57%), and the appropriate treatment instituted. Boike

63

and Graham (8) reported a stapling technique to perform an infracolic omentectomy on 13 patients. Possover et al. (9) reported 13 patients staged with ovarian cancer, Pomel et al. (10) 10 reported patients, and Spirtos et al. (11) reported four patients. Thus, 62 patients have been reported in the literature as being staged by laparoscopy, although no long-term results are available. Therefore, laparoscopy for the staging of ovarian cancer should still be considered investigational.

The two major concerns over the use of laparoscopy for adnexal masses are (i) delay in diagnosis and thus treatment, and (ii) rupture of the adnexal mass that is subsequently found to be malignant, which converts the stage from a possible IA to IC. Although studies on laparotomy show that if the tumor is removed and proper treatment instituted, rupture does not affect the outcome (12–14), it is prudent to avoid rupture to minimize any theoretical increase in the risk. If the tumor is ruptured and the treatment is delayed, the prognosis is worsened (15). Thus, the use of laparoscopy should be limited to suspicious masses that are small enough to be removed intact.

Staging of Ovarian Cancers

If an adnexal mass is found to be malignant and the operator is trained to perform staging by laparoscopy, the following conditions should be met. The mass should be ≤10 cm so that it will fit into a bag that can be removed through the vagina without spilling.

STEP 1

The para-aortic nodes should be removed to the level where the ovarian vessels originate from the vena cava on the right and the renal vein on the left.

STEP 2

Infracolic omentectomy.

STEP 3

Biopsy of the diaphragm.

STEP 4

Biopsy of the lateral colon peritoneum.

STEP 5

Inspect the bowel.

STEP 6

Remove the appendix for all mucinous tumors. It can be considered as a part of staging for the nonmucinous tumors as well.

Technique
Staging Early Ovarian Cancer

The para-aortic nodes are dissected further cephalad than is described in Chapter 2

STEP 1

The duodenum is lifted cephalad to expose the entry of the ovarian vein to the vena cava. The ureter is lateral to the ovarian vein (Fig. 6-1). The node tissue around and cephalad to the ovarian vein is removed.

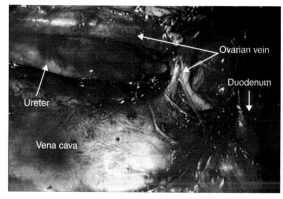

Figure 6-1. Right para-aortic nodes removed from above the ovarian vein.

STEP 2

The left para-aortic nodes are dissected above the inferior mesenteric artery. The ureter is dissected laterally and the ovarian vein is exposed where it enters the renal vein. The nodes are lifted and dissected out (Fig. 6-2).

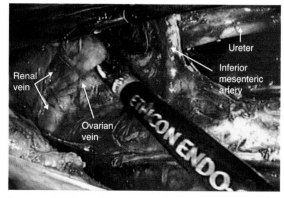

Figure 6-2. Exposing the left para-aortic nodes above the inferior mesenteric artery.

STEP 3

Omentectomy. The scope is placed in the suprapubic port. The harmonic scalpel is in the right lateral port. The assistant places traction on the omentum through the umbilical port and the left lateral port. The infracolic omentum is dissected off the transverse colon starting at the hepatic flexure (Fig. 6-3). The dissection proceeds from the right to the left until the omentum is detached. It can be removed through the vagina.

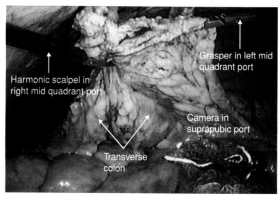

Figure 6-3. Begin omentectomy at the hepatic flexure.

STEP 4

Diaphragm biopsy. The camera is in the umbilical port or the suprapubic port. There may be small suspicious areas on the diaphragm to remove. If there are no suspicious areas, a random biopsy is performed. The harmonic scalpel or a scissor with cautery is used to make an incision in the diaphragm peritoneum. It is then peeled away (Fig. 6-4).

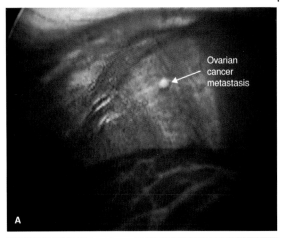

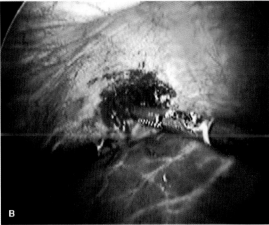

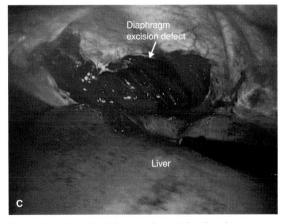

Figure 6-4. A. Nodule on the right diaphragm. **B.** Biopsy of the diaphragm. **C.** Completed excision of nodule.

STEP 5

Paracolic peritoneum. The operating table is tilted to the left to expose the right paracolic space. The peritoneum dorsal to the hepatic flexure and as high cephalad as possible is then biopsied, similar to that for the diaphragm peritoneum. The left colic peritoneum is biopsied by tilting the table to the right.

STEP 6

Appendectomy. The appendix should be removed for all mucinous tumors. It can be considered a part of staging for the other ovarian tumors as well. The mesoappendix is divided using the harmonic scalpel. Endoloops are placed over the base of the appendix and the appendix is removed by cutting between them. Irrigation is carried out.

Second-Look Laparoscopy

Laparoscopy was initially used before planned second-look laparotomy to identify residual disease and thus avoid the laparotomy. This strategy resulted in a reduction in the need for laparotomy by 50% (16).

Improvement in laparoscopic equipment has encouraged investigators to perform the entire second-look procedure by laparoscopy. Childers et al. (7) reported 44 reassessment laparoscopies in 40 women. Twenty-four of the procedures were positive, including five that were only microscopically positive. Five patients (11%) had inadequate laparoscopies due to adhesions, and recurrent disease developed in all of them. Eight of the 20 (40%) patients who were negative later had recurrent disease. All of these data were similar to those obtained with second-look laparotomy. Abu-Rustum et al. (17) reported 31 women with second-look laparoscopy and compared them with 70 patients who had laparotomy and eight who had both. The rates of positivity were 54.8%, 61.4%, and 62.5%, respectively. The recurrence rates after negative second-look were 14.8% for laparoscopy versus 14.3% for laparotomy. Clough et al. (18) reported 20 patients who had laparoscopy followed by laparotomy at the same surgery, with a positive predictive value of 86% (12 of 14 patients).

The effects of the CO_2 pneumoperitoneum and laparoscopy on the long-term survival of women undergoing second-look operations have been reported by Abu-Rustum et al. (19). During an 11-year period, there were 289 patients who had positive second-look operations. There were 131 laparoscopies using CO_2, 139 laparotomies, and 19 laparoscopies converted to laparotomy. The groups were controlled for age, stage, histology, grade, and size of disease found at second-look. The median survival for patients who had laparoscopy was 41.1 months, and for laparotomy it was 38.9 months ($p = 0.742$); thus, the overall survival was independent of the surgical approach used.

Technique

Second Look Laparoscopy

Operative Approach

Most patients will have had a large midline incision that goes around or through the umbilicus. This increases the risk of adhesions of the bowel to the umbilicus. For this reason, a direct insertion of the port into the umbilicus is not recommended. Instead, a left upper-quadrant entry is preferred.

FIGURES 5 and 6

The Verres needle is placed through a small incision between the 7th and 8th ribs in the anterior axillary line (Figs. 6-5 and 6-6). This will be 4 cm below the diaphragm. The rigidity of the ribcage allows for easy entry without countertraction on the abdominal wall. The CO_2 is insufflated to a pressure of 15 cm/pressure. The incision is enlarged to accommodate the 5-mm trocar. The trocar is then placed below the costal margin. Do not go between the ribs. The 5-mm scope is placed, and the abdomen can be inspected. If there are adhesions to the umbilicus, they are taken down by placing another 5-mm trocar in the left midquadrant and the harmonic scalpel is used to dissect the adhesions. Once the adhesions are removed from the umbilicus, a 10-mm trocar and a 10-mm trocar scope are placed.

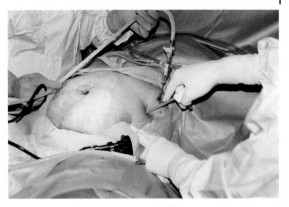

Figure 6-5. Place Verres needle between the ribs and insert the trocar below the costal margin.

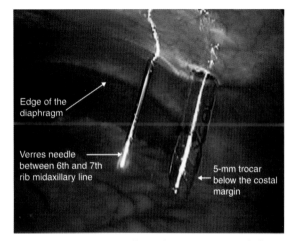

Figure 6-6. Verres needle and 5-mm trocar in left upper quadrant.

Left upper quadrant entry technique.

STEP 1

Obtain peritoneal washings for cytology. The lavage should include the diaphragm, right paracolic gutter, and pelvis.

STEP 2

Inspect the diaphragm. Biopsy any suspicious areas. If there are no suspicious areas, then remove a strip of peritoneum.

STEP 3

Biopsy any bowel adhesions.

STEP 4

Biopsy the paracolic peritoneum.

STEP 5

Biopsy the pelvic peritoneum.

STEP 6

If para-aortic nodes were not removed at the initial surgery, then they should be removed.

STEP 7

If there are remnants of the omentum, they should be biopsied.

STEP 8

The bowel should be inspected for any implants on the serosa or mesentery. Appropriate biopsies are taken.

STEP 9

If the patient has diffuse, small implants, the procedure can be terminated.

STEP 10

If the patient has tumor nodules that can be satisfactorily secondarily debulked, then a laparotomy should be performed to do that safely.

References

1. Nezhat F, Nezhat C, Welander CE, et al. Four ovarian cancers diagnosed during laparoscopic management of 1011 women with adnexal masses. *Am J Obstet Gynecol*. 1992;167:790–796.
2. Canis M, Mage G, Pouly JL, et al. Laparoscopic diagnosis of adnexal cystic masses: a 12-year experience with long-term follow-up. *Obstet Gynecol*. 1994;83:707–712.
3. Lehner R, Wenzl R, Heinzl H, et al. Influence of delayed staging laparotomy after laparoscopic removal of ovarian masses later found malignant. *Obstet Gynecol*. 1998;92:967–971.
4. Childers JM, Nasseri A, Surwit EA. Laparoscopic management of suspicious adnexal masses. *Am J Obstet Gynecol*. 1996;175:1451–1459.
5. Canis M, Pouly JL, Wattiez A, et al. Laparoscopic management of adnexal masses suspicious at ultrasound. *Obstet Gynecol*. 1997;89:679–683.
6. Querleu D, LeBlanc E. Laparoscopic infrarenal para-aortic lymph node dissection for restaging of carcinoma of the ovary or fallopian tube. *Cancer*. 1994;73:1467–1471.

7. Childers J, Lang J, Surwit E, et al. Laparoscopic surgical staging of ovarian cancer. *Gynecol Oncol*. 1995;59:25–33.

8. Boike GM, Graham JE Jr. Laparoscopic omentectomy in staging and treating gynecologic cancers. *J Am Assoc Gynecol Laparosc*. 1995;2[4 Suppl]:S4.

9. Possover M, Plaul K, Krause N, et al. Left-sided laparoscopic para-aortic lymphadenectomy: anatomy of the ventral tributaries of the infrarenal vena cava. *Am J Obstet Gynecol*. 1998;179:1295–1297.

10. Pomel C, Provencher D, Dauplat J, et al. Laparoscopic staging of early ovarian cancer. *Gynecol Oncol*. 1995;58:301–306.

11. Spirtos NM, Schlaerth JB, Spirtos TW, et al. Laparoscopic bilateral pelvic and para-aortic lymph node sampling: an evolving technique. *Am J Obstet Gynecol*. 1995;173:105–111.

12. Dembo AJ, Davy M, Stenwig AE, et al. Prognostic factors in patients with stage I epithelial ovarian cancer. *Obstet Gynecol*. 1990;75:263–273.

13. Sevelda P, Vavra N, Schemper M, et al. Prognostic factors for survival in stage I epithelial ovarian carcinoma. *Cancer*. 1990;65:2349–2352.

14. Vergote IB, Kaern J, Abeler VM, et al. Analysis of prognostic factors in stage I epithelial ovarian carcinoma: importance of degree of differentiation an deoxyribonucleic acid ploidy in predicting relapse. *Am J Obstet Gynecol*. 1993;160:40–52.

15. Maiman M, Seltzer V, Boyce J. Laparoscopic excision of ovarian neoplasms subsequently found to be malignant. *Obstet Gynecol*. 1991;77:563–565.

16. Ozols RF, Fisher RI, Anderson T, et al. Peritoneoscopy in the management of ovarian cancer. *Am J Obstet Gynecol*. 1981;140:611–619.

17. Abu-Rustum NR, Barakat RR, Siegel PL, et al. Second-look operation for epithelial ovarian cancer: laparoscopy or laparotomy? *Obstet Gynecol*. 1996;88:549–553.

18. Clough KB, Ladonne JM, Nos C, et al. Second look for ovarian cancer: laparoscopy or laparotomy? A prospective comparative study. *Gynecol Oncol*. 1999;72:411–417.

19. Abu-Rustum NR, Sonoda Y, Chi DS, et al. The effects of CO_2 pneumoperitoneum on the survival of women with persistent metastatic ovarian cancer. *Gynecol Oncol*. 2003;90:431–434.

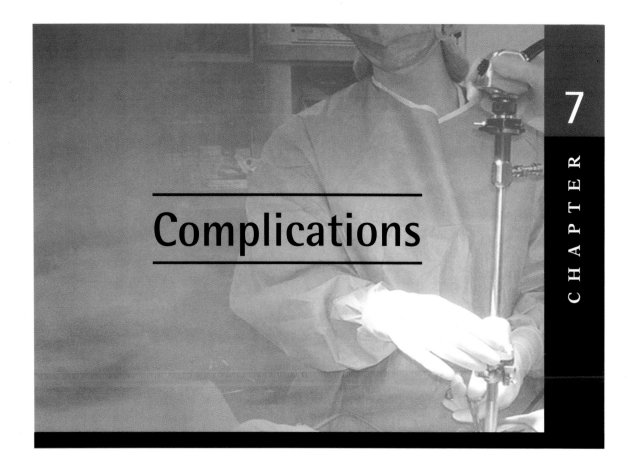

Complications

The rate of complications of laparoscopy for malignant disease is higher than those for benign disease (1). The rate depends on the type of case and the experience of the surgeon.

Electrosurgical Complications

Electrosurgery thermal injury can occur with either unipolar or bipolar instruments. The injury may occur because the tip of the electrode is in contact with bowel, bladder, or blood vessels. The zone of injury is approximately three times the observed cautery effect. Thermal injury that is recognized at the time of laparoscopy should be managed with laparotomy and excision of the injured area and closure. When monopolar electrical current is used, the patient must be adequately grounded so that the electrical current does not find a path out of the patient's body from sites other than the grounding pad, which can lead to skin burns. Modern electrosurgical units have isolated circuits with monitoring circuits that turn off the machine when the grounding pad is detached. The monopolar instruments conducting electricity should be checked for insulation defects before use. If an insulation defect comes in contact with bowel, the electrical current will exit through the bowel and cause a burn, which is usually out of the camera's view and may go unrecognized until the patient presents with peritonitis. Bipolar instruments are safer because the electricity passes between the two opposing electrodes and the only thermal effect is in the tissue that is grasped. It is recommended that the harmonic scalpel is used to avoid electrosurgical injury.

Vascular Complications

Injury to the aorta, vena cava, and common iliac vessels are the most dangerous complications. Complications occur most often with the insufflation needle, but may occur with the tip of the trocars. If blood is retrieved through the insufflation needle, the needle should be left in place while the laparotomy is being performed. Direct pressure followed by vascular surgery repair is indicated. The risk of injury to the great vessels is reduced if the insufflation needle and primary trocar are aimed toward the hollow of the sacrum at a 45-degree angle to the patient's spine. The secondary trocars should be placed under direct laparoscopic vision and angled away from the great vessels.

The inferior epigastric vessels can be avoided by proper placement of the trocars lateral to the rectus muscles (see Introduction).

Gastrointestinal Injury

The bowel may be injured by the insufflation needles, trocars, or dissection of adhesions. The risk of gastric perforation is decreased if the patient has an oral-gastric tube placed to deflate the stomach. Patients with previous midline incisions have a higher risk of injury if the trocar inserted through the umbilicus. The left upper-quadrant needle and trocar insertion is recommended in these patients. Trocar injury of the bowel is usually recognized when bowel contents and mucosa are noted as the scope is placed through the cannula. Occasionally, the trocar and cannula will completely penetrate the bowel passing through the lumen into the abdomen, and the operator will not see the bowel contents or bowel lumen. To avoid this complication, all the secondary ports should be placed under direct vision after ensuring there are no loops of bowel adhered to the abdominal wall. Primary port should be viewed through a secondary port to determine there are no loops of bowel. Injury to the stomach and bowel should be repaired with suturing; the safest way to preform this is through a small laparotomy incision. All patients have a preoperative mechanical bowel preparation, which decreases the complications from a perforation.

Enterotomy may occur any time during lysis of adhesions. Although this injury may not be apparent at the time of surgery, it does cause abdominal pain, distension, and peritonitis within 72 hours. Thermal injury that leads to perforation and peritonitis may not be diagnosed for 7 to 10 days. It is recommended that electrical instruments not be used for lysis of adhesions.

FIGURE 1

The majority of patients having laparoscopic surgery recover rapidly. If the patient is experiencing more abdominal pain, distension, and nausea after 24 hours, then an occult bowel injury should be suspected. The port sites should be inspected to determine if there is serous drainage, pus, or free air in the abdomen (Fig. 7-1). If so, an immediate laparotomy is indicated. A computed tomography scan can be performed to evaluate the amount and location of intra-abdominal air (Fig. 7-2). A small amount of air under the diaphragm is normal for the first 48 hours. There should be no gas between loops of bowel, and the liver to diaphragm separation should be no more than 3 mm.

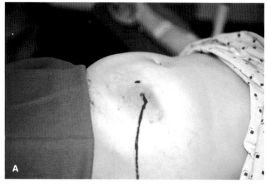

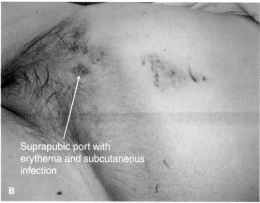

Suprapubic port with erythema and subcutaneous infection

Figure 7-1. A. Left lower quadrant trocar site with erythema, drainage and gas indicating a bowel injury. **B.** Bowel perforation causing port site infection and fistula.

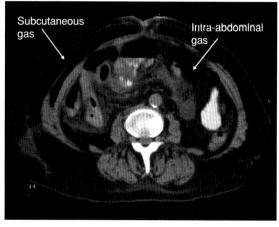

Subcutaneous gas

Intra-abdominal gas

Figure 7-2. Computed tomography scan of subcutaneous and intra-abdominal gas from bowel perforation.

Urologic Injury

The bladder may be perforated by insertion of the suprapubic trocar. Placement of a urinary catheter to deflate the bladder does not eliminate this risk. Placing the trocar at least 3 cm above the upper edge of the pubic bone is recommended. The perforations should be closed with a laparoscopic suture through the serosa and muscularis layer. Foley catheter drainage for 7 days is sufficient.

Ureteral injury may occur when dissecting pelvic endometriosis or cancer. Thermal and devascularization injuries are the most common, but they may not be discovered for up to 14 days. Typically, the patient has a fever followed by drainage of the urine through the vaginal apex. To avoid this complication, the ureter should not be touched with an active electric current.

Incisional Hernia

Herniation of omentum or bowel into the trocar sites is a complication unique to laparoscopy. Boike et al. (2) reported 19 cases from 11 institutions. No patient had a hernia through a port <10 mm; therefore, it is recommended that all port sites >10 mm be closed. Kadar et al. (3) reported a 0.17% rate of herniation among 3,560 laparoscopic operations. Occasionally, a hernia will occur at a 5-mm trocar site after a long procedure where there is significant manipulation of the cannula, which enlarges the fascial and peritoneal defects. Any 5-mm trocar site with large peritoneal or fascial openings should also be closed. The diagnosis of hernia is most often made due to pain over the trocar site. Complete obstruction of the bowel occurs when an entire loop of bowel becomes entrapped in the hernia. This will produce significantly more pain and may lead to strangulation of the bowel. The treatment is to perform an open incision over the hernia site. If the bowel is viable, it can be pushed back into the abdominal cavity and the fascia closed. If it is not viable, then a laparotomy and resection of the bowel should be undertaken.

Postoperative complications of wound infection, ileus, and fever occur, but at lower rates than after laparotomy.

References

1. Abu-Rustum N, Barakat R, Curtin J. Laparoscopic complications in gynecologic surgery for benign or malignant disease [abstract]. *Gynecol Oncol.* 1998;68:107.
2. Boike GM, Miller CE, Spirtos NM, et al. Incisional bowel herniations after operative laparoscopy: a series of nineteen cases and review of the literature. *Am J Obstet Gynecol.* 1995;172:1726–1733.
3. Kadar N, Reich H, Liu CY, et al. Incisional hernias after major laparoscopic gynecologic procedures. *Am J Obstet Gynecol.* 1993;168:1493–1495.

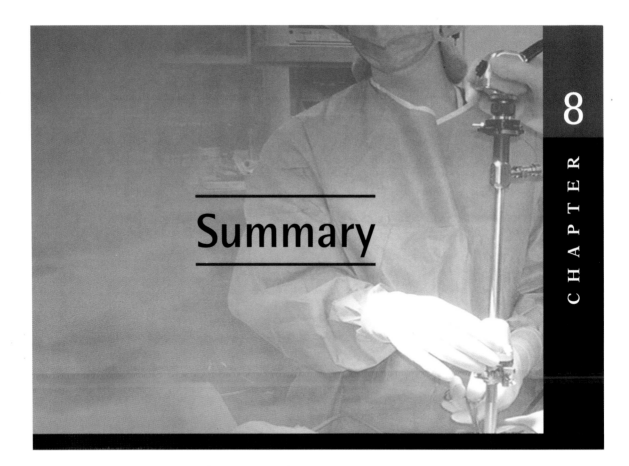

Summary

The skills to manage gynecologic malignancies by laparoscopic techniques are acquired through the surgeon's commitment to learn the technique. It requires up-to-date equipment and a team familiar with the procedures. Hands-on experience in an animal laboratory and proctored learning in the operating suite are highly recommended. In properly selected patients, laparoscopic surgery appears to result in shorter hospital stay, earlier return of function, and outcomes comparable with laparotomy, although the results of prospective, randomized trials are still to come.

Index

Note: Page numbers followed by *f* indicate figures; page numbers followed by *t* indicate tables.